The Newborn Parenting Guide (Made Easy)

Proven Methods to Stay Organized, Sleep Well & Feel Energized so You Can Find Balance & Connect with your Baby

Nicole Stanton

Medical Disclaimer

Medical disclaimer: The author is not a trained medical professional. Always consult your physician, doula, or other qualified healthcare provider for all of your medical concerns.

Table of Contents

Introduction

Becoming a parent is one of life's most exhilarating moments. Nothing beats the joy of holding your newborn in your arms for the very first time. An overwhelming sense of love has likely been bubbling inside of you since you received that positive pregnancy test result. Now that your child is here, you may have trouble finding the words to match your emotions—especially because some of those emotions aren't what you expected.

Oh, yes! Happiness, pride, and excitement fill your heart, but worry, wonder, and doubt cross your mind, too. The nursing staff at the hospital made everything look so easy, but now you're home and on your own. *How did they do that swaddle thing again? What if the baby won't latch on to feed? Did they say side-sleeping or back-sleeping was best?* These thoughts, and others like them, can put you on the verge of panic because you love this little one so much.

You might also face these other common fears:

- What if I don't know what to do?

- What if the baby stops breathing?

- What if I bump their soft spot?

- What if they won't stop crying?

- What if we can't afford everything the baby needs?

- What if we don't love them enough?

If you have stressed over things like this, you're not alone. Even if you've read all the latest books, listened to the most current podcasts, and viewed all the YouTube tutorials, you will still feel lost in your parenting journey every once in a while. That is normal, and that's okay! That's why I've created this book.

Unlike competing resources that focus on specific aspects of newborn care, this guide takes a holistic and comprehensive approach and covers a wide range of topics. You hold in your hands an in-depth guide to first-time parenting. In it, you will find quick solutions and resources to give you peace of mind and help you achieve peaceful rest, optimum health, and a deep parent-child bond. In *The Newborn Parenting Guide (Made Easy)*, you'll discover ways to tame daily challenges like those listed below:

- **Sleep deprivation:** Adjusting to interrupted sleep is one of the biggest challenges of first-time moms. You're already exhausted from nine months of pregnancy and the physical exertion of childbirth. Add to that restless nights and constant newborn care, and you're running on fumes.

- **Feeding challenges:** Determining which works best for you and your baby— breastfeeding or bottle-feeding—and managing issues like latching difficulties, low milk supply, or feeding schedules can be frustrating.

- **Postpartum recovery:** Coping with physical discomfort, healing from childbirth, managing hormonal changes, and dealing with postpartum body image concerns can sometimes lead to stress, anxiety, and depression.

- **Emotional well-being:** First-time moms often experience fluctuating emotions, postpartum mood disorders, feelings of being overwhelmed, or anxiety related to the demands of caring for a newborn.

- **Time management:** Juggling newborn care, household tasks, self-care, and potentially returning to work or managing other commitments can challenge even the most organized of moms.

- **Baby products:** The world of nursery needs is daunting. What do you need to care for your baby properly, what gadgets are helpful but unnecessary, and which items can you always leave on the store shelf?

- **Parenting advice:** Well-meaning friends and family members—and sometimes even strangers—are excited to share their experiences with new parents. But what worked for them may not work for you.

To help you navigate these and more newborn challenges, this book provides you with the following strategies:

- Instructions and tips for newborn care and parenting.

- A complete checklist of essential items you need for your newborn.

- Characteristics of a sleep-friendly environment.

- Milestones to watch for so you know if your little one is developing well.

- How to introduce siblings and pets to your newborn and vice versa.

- How to address common health issues like teething, rashes, colds, and coughs.

- Feeding advice like choosing to bottle or breastfeed and when to introduce solid foods.

- How to manage overwhelming emotions and postpartum adjustments.

You'll read real-life stories from other new parents that illustrate how to apply the advice in practical situations, and you'll find tips from experts to help you tailor your parenting approaches to your baby's unique needs.

The book adopts a straightforward, step-by-step approach to various aspects of newborn care and parenting. Each chapter is broken down into manageable portions, making implementing the strategies and recommendations easier in your daily life.

As you read, you will gain confidence in your parenting abilities. You will feel better equipped to handle challenges and make informed decisions, fostering a sense of assurance as new parents.

Chapter 1:

Preparing for Your Newborn

A baby is something you carry inside you for nine months, in your arms for three years, and in your heart till the day you die. —Mary Mason

Babies require a lot—a lot of love, a lot of attention, and a lot of stuff! It's a good thing you have about 40 weeks to prepare because it can take a while to sort through what you need and do not need. The non-essentials can also consume your energy because decorating is fun!

There are so many products available for every aspect of newborn care that just stepping into a specialty store can easily overwhelm you. From bedroom showrooms to walls of bottles, how do you know what you have to have and what you can leave on the shelf?

In this chapter, we'll sort through the must-haves, the don't-needs, and the hey-that-would-be-cools. In the appendix, you'll get checklists for furniture, bedding, feeding, diapering, clothing, storing, and more, so grab a pen or pencil and get ready! We'll also take a look at how to prepare yourself for your little one's arrival, self-care items to keep on hand, and the importance of partner support.

Setting Up the Nursery

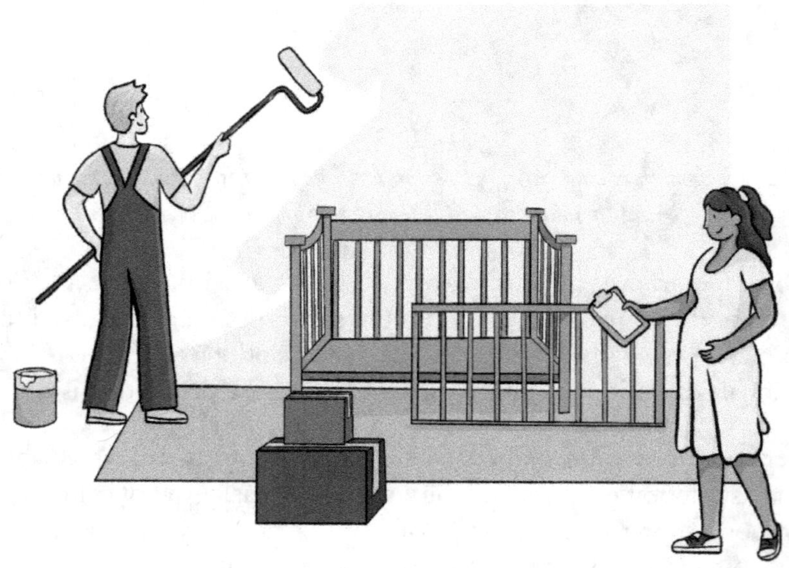

The nursery will be the biggest area in which you will do your preparations. Many questions may be running through your mind like, "Does your baby need their own room?" or "What should they have in it?"

Your Baby's Bed

Newborns sleep an average of 16 hours a day. That dwindles to about 13 hours a day by their second birthday. They nap a lot and need a safe, cozy place to do so.

The crib and bassinet are the top two choices for infant bedding. You might also find travel cribs, cradles, and boutique items like Moses' baskets, but you need a stable, secure structure in your home. Let's take a look at the pros and cons of cribs and bassinets:

- **Crib:** A traditional crib is a rectangular bedstead for babies. It has slatted, enclosed sides to keep the child from climbing out as they become bigger and more mobile. According to U.S. regulations, a standard crib mattress measures 28 inches wide by 52 inches long, slats must be no more than 2-3/8 inches apart, top rails must be at least 26 inches above the mattress, and corner posts must be no more than 1/16 of an inch above the frame. The mattress should fit so that you cannot insert anything bigger than two finger-widths between it and the rails (Chen, 2021).

    - **Pros:** Cribs are sturdy and stable and have little risk of wobbling or tipping. They can be used for several years, usually until the child is ready to transition to a regular bed. Crib size is regulated and standardized, making it easy to find mattresses, sheets, and mattress pads to fit your piece of furniture. You can adjust the mattress level to grow with your child, and some cribs convert into toddler or twin beds, saving you money down the road.

    - **Cons:** Cribs can be expensive. Their size and bulk can be cumbersome if your home has limited space. It can be challenging to place the baby into a crib or lift them back out.

- **Bassinet:** A bassinet is a small bed designed for babies from birth to four months of age, weigh about 20 pounds, or can roll over on their own. Bassinets are often oval-shaped with mesh sides and can be moved easily.

    - **Pros:** Bassinets are much easier to place your baby into and get them back out of. This is especially helpful for women who've had a C-section and have difficulty bending and reaching. Bassinets are also portable, so you can move them from room to room and keep your baby nearby. The smaller, more mobile bassinet fits into even small rooms, and some double as a bedside sleeper. They are also less expensive than cribs.

- ○ **Cons:** While it may save upfront expenses, bassinets are temporary. Your baby will outgrow it quickly, and you will still need to purchase a crib later on. If your baby is active, or if you have curious pets, your bassinet may tip, so you need to monitor it when it's in use.

The American Academy of Pediatrics (AAP) confirms that cribs and bassinets are safe options. They do recommend using a tightly fitted sheet over a mattress pad and to follow the below recommendations (Blackman, 2020):

- Place your baby on their back to sleep; never put them facedown.

- Avoid using sleep positioners or other sleep aids for your baby.

- Do not use crib bumpers.

- Remove all loose items like blankets, plush toys, or clothing from your baby's sleeping area.

- Have your child sleep in the same room with you until they are at least six months old.

- Do not sleep with the baby in your bed.

- Do not attach mobiles to the crib or bassinet.

- Don't place the crib or bassinet near a window where they could pull on blinds, strings, or curtains.

- Make sure the crib mattress is no more than six inches thick.

- Purchase your crib or bassinet new to be sure it meets the most current safety standards.

Ultimately, the choice of bedstead is up to you. Just follow the manufacturer's assembly instructions so that everything is put together securely and follow the above safety tips, and your baby will have a comfy, cushy place to rest.

Nursery Furnishings and Decor

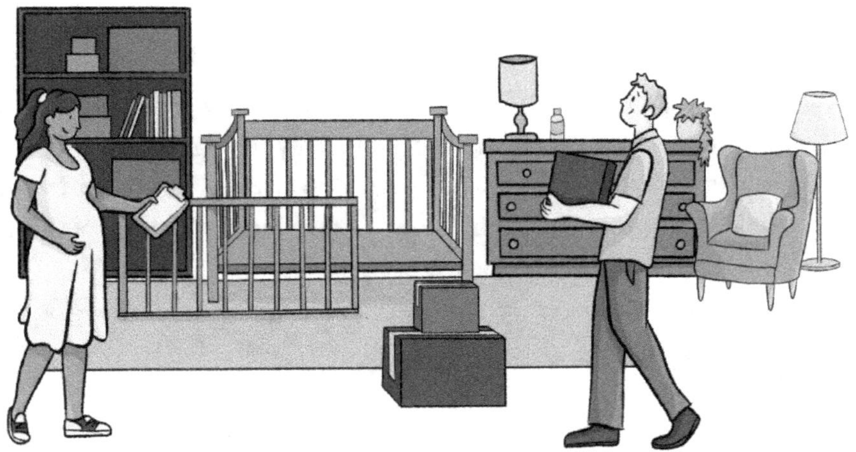

Once you've chosen your baby's bed and gotten it set up, you'll need some other furnishings for comfort and organization. The below items are must-haves, but you can be creative with the styles you choose:

- **Rocking chair or glider:** This one's for you, Mom and Dad! Every new parent needs a comfortable chair in the nursery. Yes, the rocking motion helps soothe the baby, but it also calms you. A rocker or glider is the perfect place to nurse or bottle feed, hum a lullaby, whisper a bedtime story, or just cuddle.

- **Changing table with pad:** You can purchase a changing table designed specifically for diapering and organization or select a dresser or other furniture item that has a temporary changing station built-in that can be removed when it's no longer needed. Most come with a pad, but if yours doesn't have one, you can purchase one separately. Be sure to get the right size that fits snugly into its space.

- **Chest of drawers, dresser, or other clothes storage option:** Babies go through so much clothing, so you need a place to store it all. Often, because they're so tiny, newborn items can be arranged on the shelves of a changing table. But, eventually, you'll need something more substantial, like a stable chest of drawers. Another option is to place storage bins or an organizer in the closet. This frees up space in the room, and the closet doors can be shut and secured to keep the child from getting into things as they grow.

- **Hanging or wall shelves:** In this chapter, we focus on what you *need* for your new baby, but let's face it, you're going to have many nonessentials too. You can find decorative wall shelves in various styles, like ones that hang from the ceiling, secure to the wall, or stand alone. Shelves make great displays and keep things out of reach of little fingers when your child is bigger and more mobile.

Note: As your child grows, they may pull on or attempt to climb on furniture. To prevent falling over and injury to your baby, secure the dresser or chest of drawers, standing shelves, changing table, and other pieces of furniture to a wall stud. Most new items come with ties attached to the back, but you can also purchase the accessories separately.

Essential Soft Goods to Have in the Nursery

All the necessary furnishings are in your baby's room. It looks good but a little bare, isn't it? Let's make it more inviting by bringing in some cozy comforts.

In the first section, we assessed your choice of bedstead: crib or bassinet. Whether you've chosen one or both options, you'll need to make it comfortable and sleep-ready. Here are some things you'll need:

- **Waterproof pads:** Crib and bassinet mattresses are usually water-resistant; however, diapers sometimes leak, and it's convenient to replace the pad when you have an issue. Waterproof pads are sold in full crib sizes or smaller varieties that work well with bassinets and other bedding options. Be sure to place the pad under the fitted sheet, not over it.

- **Fitted sheets:** Sheets are sold to fit specific mattress sizes. Cribs are standardized unless you purchase one with a custom shape, so sheeting is usually easy to find. For bassinets and other bedstead options, purchase only what fits your mattress measurements. Loose sheets can pose a suffocation hazard and increase risk of sudden infant death syndrome (SIDS).

Some other items you'll need in the baby's room include changing table pad covers, receiving blankets, burp cloths, bibs, bath towels, washcloths, and a nursing pillow. Blackout window curtains are not essential, but they are helpful to prevent unwanted light from disturbing the baby's sleep or waking them too soon.

Swaddle blankets are also a popular but nonessential purchase. Many parents find that when they bind their baby this way, the baby feels secure, like when they were in the womb, and rests more peacefully. Swaddling also controls their motions, so involuntary movements like flailing arms or legs won't startle them awake. Here's how to properly swaddle your baby:

1. Spread out the blanket on a flat surface and place it on the diamond angle. Then, fold down the top corner about six inches.

2. Lay the baby on their back, ensuring their shoulders are at the folded edge.

3. Gently place the baby's left arm down by their side and pull the corner of the blanket on that side over the baby's body, tucking it under their right side.

4. Loosely lay the bottom corner of the blanket over the baby's feet and legs. *Note*: Make sure their legs can freely bend up and out and are not tightly bound inside the blanket! Their legs should

be able to spread apart naturally, and their hips should be able to rotate out and around.

5. Gently place the baby's right arm down by their side and pull the blanket across their body, tucking it under their back.

6. To ensure it's not wrapped too tightly, check to see that you can get at least two fingers between your baby's chest and the blanket.

Note: Always place your baby on their back to sleep—especially when swaddled—to reduce the risk of SIDS.

Your Baby's Wardrobe

Clothing is definitely essential! Infants can be messy. Between feedings, spit-up, and leaky diapers, they may go through several outfits a day. Keeping clothes organized and within reach of the changing table is smart.

Some pieces that should be in every baby's wardrobe are onesies, pajamas, and socks. Onesies are soft, cotton t-shirts that secure at the bottom. They come in many colors and prints, are inexpensive, and can be worn alone or under other clothing. Though onesies are cute and convenient, they should not be worn overnight. Children's nightwear is specially treated to be flame retardant to protect them in the event of a fire, so be sure to purchase jammies, sleepers, or sleeping sacks for bedtime. Baby socks are notorious for falling off or being kicked off when they bump their feet together, but keeping those tiny toes warm is essential.

Only buy a few of any particular size. Babies grow quickly and can grow out of a favorite outfit within days, so always keep the next size handy. The appendix in the back of the book gives you an idea of clothes you should have in the baby's room. If you live in a warm climate, you might not need some of the wintery items, but you should at least layer your baby's clothes or have a sweater or jacket ready for cooler days.

Feeding, Diapering, and Bathing

These three things will consume your days, at least during the first few months. Whether you choose to breastfeed or bottle feed, you'll need to have certain supplies available, like bottles, nipples in different sizes, bottle cleaners, sterilizers, and organizers. If you're nursing, you'll need a breast pump and milk storage bags or containers; if you're bottle feeding, you'll need formula. In a later chapter, we'll discuss feeding options in-depth, but it's wise to stock up on necessities now.

Keeping your baby's bottom clean and dry will not only keep them happy and comfortable, but it will also prevent irritation, rashes, and infections. Babies go through countless diapers each day—up to 3,000 during their first year—so be sure to buy more than you think you'll need. If you go with disposables, have at least two boxes on hand, and keep the next size up available.

In general, disposable diaper sizes are as follows: preemie (under 6 pounds), newborn (up to 10 pounds), size 1 (8-14 pounds), size 2 (12-18 pounds). size 3 (16-28 pounds), size 4 (22-37 pounds), size 5 (over 27 pounds), and size 6 (over 35 pounds). Some children may be bigger at birth than others and skip the newborn size altogether. As your due date approaches, see if your doctor can provide an estimated birth weight.

If you choose to use cloth diapers, purchase multiple packs as well as several waterproof covers. You'll also need lots of wipes or cleansing cloths, a diaper pail with lots of liners, and rash cream just in case it's needed. Furthermore, remember to stock your diaper bag for when you're on the go!

Most babies enjoy bath time. It can be very calming and soothing, and it helps them relax. When your infant is a newborn, you'll want to bathe them in a portable tub. You can place the tub in a large, clean kitchen sink or set it inside the bathtub. Its small size makes handling the baby more convenient, and it will keep the baby from slipping. You will need a gentle baby soap and shampoo, washcloths, hooded towels, and as they get a bit bigger, age-appropriate tub toys to keep them occupied while you wash their little bodies. An optional bath visor is helpful to keep soapy water from dripping down your child's face and into their eyes.

Car Seats, Toys, Storage, and More

A lot of baby needs are simply a matter of preference. Many, like cribs and mattresses, must meet safety standards, but one nursery necessity is required by law: the infant car seat. You cannot leave the hospital without one that meets legal requirements and that is correctly installed in your vehicle.

An infant car seat should be installed in the rear-facing position in the backseat of your vehicle. It is recommended that children travel in the rear-facing position as long as possible. Your baby will likely outgrow the height and weight limits of their infant seat within their first year. At that point, you should purchase a convertible or all-in-one seat that will fit them much longer. Once your child surpasses the maximum height and weight requirements (between the ages 1–3) for the rear-facing seat, they may switch to forward-facing. Again, adhere to your car seat's recommendations and keep your child in the protective seat until they are big enough to fit safely in a booster (usually between the ages 4–7). When they are big enough to sit in the vehicle and have the seatbelt hold them in proper position (between the ages 8–12), they will no longer need the booster; however, they will still be safer in the back seat (NHTSA, n.d.).

Other miscellaneous items you'll want to include are a sturdy stroller, infant swing, bouncer seat, and a portable crib. It's also convenient to have a baby monitor—with or without video—so you can hear when your napping baby begins to stir or cry out. Night-lights, storage bins, toys, and household baby proofing items should also be on your checklist.

Designing a Soothing Space

You've assembled all the furnishings and collected all the necessities you'll need for your baby's first few weeks and months. Now, what are you going to do with them? You'll want everything to be accessible, but you don't want the baby's space to be crowded or cramped. Ideally, it would be best to aim for a balance of form and function that creates a soothing space for your little one and is organized for maximum utility.

When creating a calming nursery, consider the following tips:

- **Paint the walls in soft colors, like neutral tones and pale blues and greens, to create a relaxing atmosphere.** Soft colors won't overstimulate your baby like bright, primary colors do.

- **Have a variety of textures in the room.** Fluffy teddy bears, velvety curtains, and plush blankets provide a pleasant sensory experience with a calming effect.

- **Make it comfy for you too.** You'll be spending a lot of time in the nursery, rocking your child, changing diapers, playing, and bonding together. Keep a cozy blanket in the rocker with your nursing pillow to make the space relaxing and inviting for both you and your child.

- **Play peaceful sounds to help your baby and you feel more at ease.** White noise machines or apps that play soothing music can help your baby associate the sound with sleep time and help them drift back to sleep if they wake in the night.

- **Don't crowd the space.** Keep diapers, toys, clothing, and other essentials put away and organized so there is open space in the room. This also allows for tummy time and play area as your child grows.

- **Dim the lights.** Low-wattage lamps and nightlights—particularly lights that mimic natural outdoor light—make the nursery seem warm and inviting as well as promote restful sleep.

- **Put storage bins under the crib.** This works really well for diapers and wipes during the first few months, and it makes a great place to keep toys as your child becomes mobile.

- **Use storage organizers to keep everything in place and out of the way.** Place dividers in dresser drawers to separate clothing items. Use clothespins to attach shirts or pants to regular-size hangers to avoid purchasing baby-sized ones. Attach changeable signs to the hanging bar in the closet to keep clothes separated by size and use an over-the-door shoe organizer for baby shoes and booties, sun hats, mittens, or other small items.

Once everything is arranged and ready for the baby, take some time to get yourself ready for their arrival.

Preparing Yourself for Your Baby's Arrival

We've talked a lot about preparing the nursery, but there are some things you need to do to prepare *yourself* for your baby's arrival as well.

Taking Care of Yourself

Self-care is trendy. Open any social media platform, and you'll find numerous suggestions on how to pamper yourself. However, you shouldn't take the subject lightly when you are expecting. Your body has already been through many changes, and it still has a lot of work to do to complete your pregnancy, like delivering your little one and recovering. Treat your body kindly and give it some TLC. Your overall well-being will improve, and you'll be more confident to face the days ahead.

Below are some helpful ways to prepare yourself for your baby's arrival:

- **Detach from technology one full day each week.** If you're worried your friends will think something's wrong, let them know in advance that you'll be unplugging and won't be checking in.

- **Take 5–15 minutes a day to do what you enjoy.** It's not a time to catch up on work or finish organizing the baby's closet. Choose an activity that calms you and brings you peace, like reading, painting, or listening to music.

- **If you are a person of faith or are spiritually inclined, study religious texts, pray, or connect with others who share your beliefs.** You may also repeat affirmations and mantras.

- **Keep a journal of your thoughts and experiences.** You could also devote it to gratitude and note something you are thankful for each day. You can also do a brain dump in your journal. Set a timer for 15 minutes and write down whatever is on your mind. Address anything urgent and note the other things to be handled later.

- **Enjoy light exercise like stretching or yoga that's appropriate for your pregnancy stage.** Include breathing exercises, and when you can, sit or lie down with your eyes closed to ensure you're getting enough rest.

- **Ask your spouse or partner to help with household tasks.** This includes having them help you prep the nursery.

- **Talk to your partner.** Nurture the connection you have and strengthen your bond. Both of you are anxious, so use the time to talk about your concerns and grow together as you get closer to becoming parents.

- **Tend to your physical needs too.** Stay hydrated, eat a balanced diet, maintain personal hygiene, stay active, get a good night's rest, and replace beauty items that contain harsh chemicals with ones that are gentler on your skin. Keep the below checklist handy and make sure you have the necessary items for your postnatal care when you bring your baby home from the hospital.

Give yourself compassionate care. You'll have more self-confidence and higher self-esteem, and you'll feel more prepared to embrace parenthood.

How to Prepare Yourself Emotionally for Parenthood

Becoming a parent is a significant change. Every aspect of your life will be different from this point forward. You are now a family, and while your carefree days of impromptu outings may be a thing of the past, you'll soon find that days filled with preparation and planning can make your new normal just as exciting—if not more so, since now you'll have your child to make your life complete.

This is a big transition. We've talked a lot about preparing the nursery, but how can you prepare yourself emotionally for parenthood? Below is some helpful advice:

- **Slow down while you can.** Once the baby arrives, your world may become chaotic as you adjust to meeting their needs on a severe sleep shortage, working around a seemingly never-ending stream of well-meaning visitors, and patiently allowing your body to heal from all it has gone through. Rest now, practice the self-care tips outlined above, and take advantage of your downtime.

- **Have realistic expectations.** It's wonderful to set goals and work toward being the best parent you can be, but know that there is no such thing as a perfect parent and no one right way to parent. You will find your unique groove, which may look much different than your best friend's.

- **Try not to compare yourself to others, especially not to social media influencers who post nothing but picture-perfect ideals.** Embrace the fact that you will have good days and bad. The good won't make you the best, but the bad won't make you the worst. Together, however, they will make you the perfect parent for your child.

- **Establish your support network now.** There are lots of possibilities. The first place to look is to those closest to you, like grandparents, aunts, uncles, and best friends. You don't have to follow everyone's advice, but it's nice to hear about the experiences of those who've gone before you to know you're not alone in this newness. Advice from your support network also gives you a chance to discover tips and tricks you hadn't thought of before. Community support groups are also great places to connect with other first-time parents. You'll find just the right connections in these or hobby and special interest groups, church or community support groups, and virtual or online groups.

Partner Involvement

Parenthood changes everything, especially your relationship with your spouse or partner. Stress, worry, and lack of sleep can put you both on edge in the days leading up to delivery and in the first few days and weeks after your child is born. The two of you are in new roles now, and adjusting takes time. Remember that you created a child together, so you are crazy about each other! Hold on to that perspective and support each other with kindness and compassion.

Men don't talk as much about it as much as women do, but both of you have likely had your share of worries stack up. Concerns about your health during your pregnancy, your baby's health, the pending delivery and childbirth experience, the future, and much more can overwhelm both of you mentally and emotionally. Once your child arrives, you might find that you are bonding with the baby but struggling to nurture the bond you have with each other.

Know that you are not alone! You and your partner are in this together. You have each other as a built-in support system. Date night might look different now. It may consist of a candlelit bowl of cereal at the kitchen table, but make that moment matter. Show each other physical affection with a back rub or cuddle, and always keep the lines of communication open. Make the time you share meaningful.

In Summary

This chapter focused on preparing to welcome your new baby into your home and life. We looked at furnishings, soft goods, organizers, and feeding needs, as well as how to create a welcoming environment for your child to come home to and how to prepare yourself for this new journey you're embarking on.

When you shop for necessities, take this book and a pen or pencil with you and mark the checklists. Note which items you've already purchased or received as gifts so you don't duplicate things—and remember the self-care items!

As we move forward, we'll discuss bringing your new baby home, newborn sleeping essentials, feeding options, and how to bond with your baby.

Chapter 2:

The First Days and Weeks

The moment a child is born, the mother is also born. She never existed before. The woman existed, but the mother, never. A mother is something absolutely new. —
Bhagwan Shree Rajneesh

Congratulations! Your baby has been born, and things are flowing smoothly. Your new little one is on a great sleeping and feeding schedule. You're getting lots of rest. Someone else is doing all the cooking and cleaning. Parenthood is a breeze! Well, it is until you leave the hospital.

The nurses' round-the-clock help teased you and set you up for false expectations. Now that you're home, things are a bit chaotic. Everyone wants to stop by to see the baby at any time on any day, you and the baby are trying to figure each other out, and sleep is a distant memory. The good news is that you *can* find your groove if you take things one day at a time.

In this chapter, you will discover how to transition from hospital to home with ease. We'll also talk about how to help your infant get to sleep (and stay asleep), introduce feeding methods, and look at ways you and your partner can bond with your baby.

Bringing Baby Home

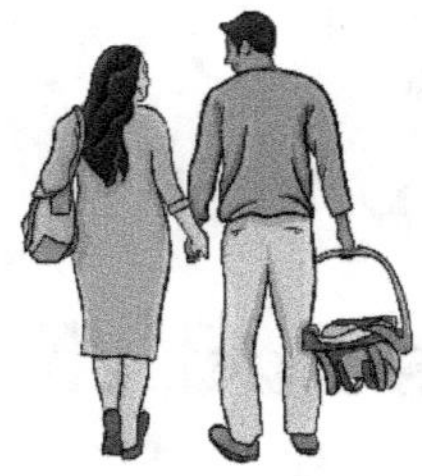

Going home from the hospital is an exciting time, whether that happens right away or after a medically necessary stay. There are certain things a new parent needs to know about bringing a baby home.

What to Wear... or Not

New parents often choose a special "going home" outfit for their newborn to wear when they leave the hospital, and sometimes moms have a special new dress for themselves as well. Cute clothes can make you feel good! They can also provide great photo ops and announcement images to share with friends and family or to print and frame.

Don't overdo it, though. Newborns aren't used to being handled very much yet, and they're also not used to wearing clothes. Choose an outfit that is made of a soft material, is lightweight, and is easy to get on and off. Something bulky, scratchy, or requires you to manipulate their arms and legs a lot while dressing them can make them uncomfortable and upset.

Also, take note of the weather. If it's warm, a dress or a T-shirt with pants will do just fine. Then, simply place a light blanket over your baby's legs for the car ride home, being sure to keep the blanket down and away from the child's face. If it's cold outside, dress them in a long-sleeved, full-body outfit with foot coverings, or put socks or booties on them. Also, be sure to place a knit cap on their head, and, again, cover their legs with a blanket.

Moms, whether you have something new to wear or not, be sure whatever you pack is loose-fitting and a couple sizes up from your pre-pregnancy size. An oversized T-shirt and stretchy pants or a flowy dress are ideal options. Remember to also pack breastfeeding-friendly clothes with buttons or tops made specifically for this purpose.

Is Your Baby Ready to Go Home?

Before you go home, specific requirements must be met regarding your child's health. The attending doctor or other hospital staff will check to see if your baby meets the following conditions:

- Your baby has taken at least two successful feedings.

- Your baby has had at least one wet diaper and passed at least one bowel movement.

- Your baby's temperature is normal.

- Your baby is not jaundiced or at risk of developing jaundice.

- Your baby has been given any necessary vaccines and medications.

- Your baby has been administered any required screenings or tests.

If you delivered your baby prematurely, in addition to the above, doctors will check for the following criteria:

- Your baby's breathing is strong and clear.

- Your baby hasn't lost a substantial amount of weight since birth or is steadily gaining an appropriate amount.

- Depending on the circumstances surrounding the preterm birth, your baby may be screened for hearing impairment or given other tests.

Although you are probably anxious to get home and begin this new adventure, don't feel rushed to leave the hospital. If you'll be breastfeeding, make sure you're comfortable with the process. Know the signs of complications that could arise. Ask whatever questions you have before you go home.

Note: Premature births and other complications may require newborns, and sometimes women who have just given birth, to remain in the hospital for additional treatment and care. This, of course, may alter the requirements that must be met before either can be released from the medical facility.

The Car Ride Home

As mentioned in Chapter 1, a rear-facing infant car seat is required by law to be installed in your vehicle for the drive home. *Never ride in any vehicle without properly restraining your child, and never install a car seat in the front passenger seat!* Both of these actions could result in severe injury and death in the event of an accident.

You can choose between the below car seat options:

- **Infant-only:** These small, portable, rear-facing-only seats are designed for newborns and infants. Your child will outgrow it when they get to about 22-35 pounds, so you will need to purchase the larger convertible seat. Always adhere to the weight and height standards from the manufacturer before moving your child into a bigger or different seat. Infant car seats have a convenient carry handle, and some can attach to a stroller for an easy transition when traveling with your baby.

- **Convertible:** Even if you choose to skip the infant seat and go straight to the convertible seat, it still needs to face the back of the vehicle until your child is at least two years old or has reached the maximum height and weight requirements as stated by the manufacturer, whichever comes first.

In either case, buying new is preferred so that you know its true condition and can register with the manufacturer, which will allow you to receive recalls or other notifications. If you borrow or purchase a used seat, check the expiration date on the seat and do not buy it if it is six years old or older, as the materials may no longer hold up in the event of an accident. Also, ensure a preowned seat has not been involved in a car accident, shows no signs of cracks or other wear and tear, and is not missing any components.

If you are unsure how to properly install your baby's car seat, many hospitals, police stations, and fire stations are happy to assist and check the security of its positioning.

Going Home With Mixed Feelings

It's common to focus on the romantic aspects of having a baby. Still, sometimes in that joy, you overlook and under-anticipate the toll that pregnancy, childbirth, and recovery take on your physical and emotional states.

For about 40 weeks, your hormones were in flux and still are. Your frame strained to support additional weight, which you will carry a little while longer. Plus, you were and still are tired all the time. You were hungry, nauseous, happy, and sad, and now that the baby's here, all these things may converge on you at once.

While you're overjoyed to finally hold your baby in your arms, you may also struggle with uncertain feelings like those below:

- **You are experiencing depression and feel overloaded or overwhelmed by the need to meet your baby's needs.** Not to mention, you are also tending to your own recovery while maintaining your home, taking care of other children you may have, and being an affectionate partner to your spouse. Such feelings, commonly referred to as the "baby blues," typically go away on their own within a couple weeks. However, if they are not addressed and do not resolve quickly, you may develop a more severe condition called postpartum depression, which we'll discuss in a later chapter.

- **You feel anxious and have a sense of hyper-vigilance, which keeps you on high alert.** You experience panic attacks as a result of being in such an exaggerated state of intensity.

- **You may feel nervous, especially if this is your first child.** Even though you have prepared yourself by reading all the experts' books and watching all the latest tutorials, you may still worry that you won't know what to do or be able to adequately meet your child's needs.

- **You may be upset by your baby's crying, which sometimes seems to go on without end.** It's helpful to remember that newborns cry for 1–5 hours within a 24-hour period, but the amount of crying will slowly subside as weeks progress. It's really the only way they can let you know they need you at this stage.

All these feelings are normal and valid. You are not a bad parent for having doubts. You're a loving and attentive parent for having these concerns and wanting to ensure you always meet your child's needs.

Newborn Sleep Essentials

We spent a lot of time in Chapter 1 on setting up the nursery and preparing a comfortable space for your new baby. Now that your newborn is here, it's time to put those arrangements to work.

Experts used to recommend keeping the baby's room bright and appealing to the senses. They encouraged light, color, and decorations that stimulated the baby's brain. New studies, however, have shown that dim light, soft colors, and minimal decorations calm babies and improve their sleep (*Sleep Guide*, n.d.). When they sleep better, so do you, so let's take a look at other tips to support your baby's sound sleep.

Below is a list of ways to create a sleep-friendly environment for your baby:

- **Dim the lights:** During wakeful play time, turn on the overhead light, open the curtains, and let in the sun to encourage activity, but at sleep time, shut it all down. Light delays the release of melatonin, taking it longer for your baby's brain to signal it to rest. If you keep a nightlight on, use a bulb in the red-orange spectrum. Invest in blackout curtains if you don't already have them and keep them closed during naps and overnight.

- **Turn down the noise:** Quiet calms the brain. Turn off noisy toys, televisions, and other devices that could keep your baby awake. You could utilize a white noise machine or app to block out other sounds in the house from disturbing the baby's sleep. It should be no louder than 50 decibels (about the volume of a running shower) and should be placed across the room from the baby's bed.

- **Keep it cool:** Lower room temperatures lead to fewer sleep interruptions. As Rockin' Blinks explains (*Sleep Guide*, n.d.), the human body temperature changes throughout the day. It is warmest about one to two hours before bedtime and drops rapidly once asleep. It remains low until about an hour or two before it's time to wake up. The cooler temperature enables sleep by slowing metabolism and reducing alertness. Room temperatures should ideally be between 68°F and 72°F. Rooms that are too warm have been shown to increase the occurrence of SIDS.

- **Follow safety standards:** Review the safety protocols mentioned in the previous chapter regarding crib and mattress measurements, placement, and anchoring. Also, remember to keep loose items like blankets and toys out of the baby's bed while they sleep to reduce suffocation, choking, and SIDS. As your child gets bigger, they may climb out of their bed, so have child-proofing items installed throughout the house to ensure they can't harm themselves if they wander during the night.

On top of making the room comfortable, try the below suggestions to help your baby fall asleep and stay asleep longer:

- **Have a consistent routine:** Keeping to a regular schedule will help the baby learn that certain times of the day are for staying awake and others are for sleeping. Their bodies will soon learn to tire and become restful as their circadian rhythm adapts to the routine.

- **Swaddle your baby:** Swaddling keeps the baby tucked in and feeling secure. If you haven't mastered the swaddle fold, don't worry! You can purchase a ready-wrap version or tuck the baby into a sleep sack. Make sure it's not too tight and that the baby's hips and legs are free to move.

- **Place the baby on their back to sleep:** This is the safest sleeping position. It significantly reduces the risk of SIDS and allows for easy breathing.

- **Consider a humidifier:** If you live in an arid environment or have noticeably drier air during the winter months, a cool-mist humidifier can reduce dryness and discomfort. Clean it regularly to keep it free from bacteria and mold.

We'll take a more in-depth look at sleep challenges and successes in Chapter 4.

Newborn Feeding Essentials

Your new little one needs nourishment, of course, and there are only two choices for the first few months: breast or bottle. Some people have strict opinions on this matter, but the important point is to choose what is right for *you and your child*.

Statistics show that around 80% of newborns are breastfed, and approximately half are still being nursed at six months, but only one third continue after that age (Porter, 2018). While "breast is considered best" because it contains all the nutrition your baby needs, formula is an excellent alternative when breastfeeding is not an option.

Some benefits of breastfeeding include the following (Porter, 2018):

- Its nutrients encourage brain growth, improve eye function, and further develop the nervous system.

- It's automatically heated to the right temperature because your breasts can detect as little as a single degree variation in your baby's body temperature.

- It reduces the risk of SIDS.

Some benefits of bottle-feeding include the following:

- It allows your spouse or other caregivers to take part in the feeding and bonding.

- Some bottle-fed babies sleep through the night sooner than breastfed ones because they stay fuller longer.

- It allows you to heal if you have pain, infection, or other difficulties with breastfeeding.

There's a lot to consider when choosing your child's feeding method. Your top priority is to make sure they're receiving a sufficient amount of nutrients and vitamins. We will take a comprehensive look at how, when, and what to feed your newborn in the next chapter.

Bonding and Communication

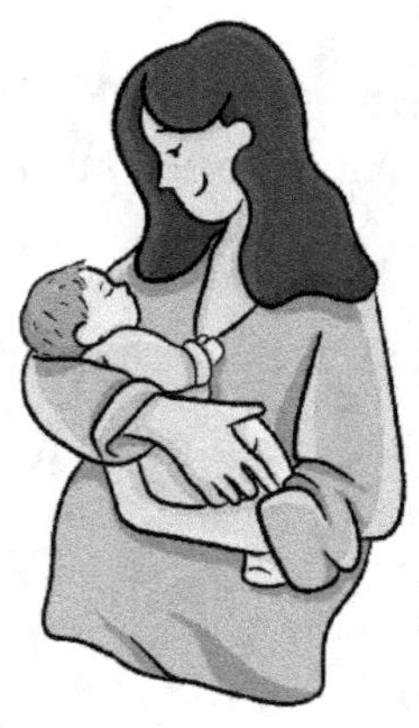

Before your child is born, you will likely experience strong feelings of love for your infant. This love doesn't need to be proven or reciprocated! It's innate, and it intensifies once your baby arrives. It's not based on needs, and it has no conditions. It's the affection and desire to share a unity with your baby that stems from your natural urge to care for your child. This is bonding.

Bonding is the connection that forms between you and your child, and it is an integral part of becoming a parent. While the term is often used interchangeably with "attachment," the two concepts differ. Bonding is directed from the parent toward the child, and attachment is from the child toward the parent. Both require intimacy, physical touch, and quality interactions, and both of you benefit from similar behaviors.

Bonding is essential because it helps the baby trust you, know they can rely on you to tend to them, and securely attach to you. Skin-to-skin contact is a great way to establish your bond from the start and nurture that connection in the early days and weeks.

What Is Skin-To-Skin Contact?

Skin-to-skin contact, sometimes referred to as "kangaroo care," first occurs immediately after birth, when the baby is dried and placed on the mother's unclothed chest. Both are covered to stay warm and are allowed to remain in this closeness for at least an hour until the first feeding or as long as the mother desires, if neither the baby nor the mother is in distress or needs medical attention. It has become the standard practice in delivery rooms since Dr. Philip Sunshine introduced the idea in the 1960s.

In the '60s, Sunshine, emeritus professor of pediatrics at Lucile Packard Children's Hospital Stanford and a creator of modern neonatal care, studied the effects of skin-to-skin contact with babies born preterm. Among the benefits, Sunshine (n.d.) discovered that the mother's release of oxytocin, also known as the "love hormone," soothes and calms both mother and child, stimulates the milk supply, and helps the uterus contract.

Some other benefits of skin-to-skin contact include the following:

- It strengthens the baby's heart.

- It improves the baby's lung function.

- It stabilizes the mother's and the baby's body temperatures.

- It reduces the newborn's crying.

- It relieves post-delivery pain for both mother and child.

- It regulates the baby's blood glucose.

- It introduces friendly bacteria to the baby's skin.

It is highly recommended for your husband or partner to participate in skin-to-skin time as well. In this way, the baby learns the scents and feel of their other parent, allowing them to form a healthy attachment with both parents.

You can continue skin-to-skin contact beyond the newborn stage by making adjustments as your child grows. Pats on the back or gentle shoulder rubs can have similar soothing effects and help keep your bond secure.

Understanding Your Baby's Communication by Reading Their Cues

Communication is imperative for effectively meeting your infant's needs. But, how do you know what they're telling you? *Is your baby hungry? Tired? Wet?* You will gradually learn to recognize variations in the tone, volume, and urgency of your newborn's cries, but there are other cues that will help you more fully understand your child's message—it just takes a little time and patience.

Below are some ways your baby communicates with you, grouped by what they're trying to say:

- **Your baby is ready to interact:**

  - The baby is awake and alert.

  - The baby's eyes are wide and searching for a friendly face.

  - The baby brings their hand to the side of their face, mouth, or ear.

  - The baby tucks their feet up to the middle of their body.

  - The baby moves in smooth, not startled motions.

- **Your baby needs a break:**

  - The baby is fussy or crying lightly.

  - The baby's body is tense and stiff or very limp and tired.

  - The baby is restless, squirmy, and unsettled.

  - The baby arches their back or pushes their hand out toward you with a stiff arm.

  - The baby won't make eye contact and turns away.

- **Your baby is hungry:**

  - The baby licks or smacks their lips.

  - The baby sucks on whatever comes near their mouth.

  - The baby will lift up their head.

  - The baby will root around your breasts or the chest of the person holding them.

  - The baby will be fussy and may cry in short, low pitches.

- **Your baby is tired:**

  - The baby will cry and be fussy.

  - The baby will press their lips together, frown, or have a dull expression.

  - The baby's skin may pale.

  - The baby may breathe more rapidly.

  - The baby may look away.

Once you get to know your infant's signals and sounds, you'll gain confidence in your parenting skills and take comfort in knowing you are meeting your child's needs well.

Stimulating Your Baby's Development Through Play

Your baby will grow both physically and cognitively very quickly during their first few months. They will achieve a lot of developmental milestones by the time they are six months old, like responding when they hear their name spoken, responding to familiar voices, turning toward sounds, smiling in response to attention, and babbling.

According to Nationwide Children's Hospital, below are some target gains you can look forward to (*Developmental Milestones*, n.d.):

- **Birth to 3 months**: Your baby will learn to turn their head to the side and lift it briefly while lying on their belly.

- **Three months**: Your baby will be able to bring their hands together and raise them to their mouth, kick their legs when they lie on their back, swipe their hands and arms toward a toy, shake a rattle, and sit with support.

- **From 3 to 4 months:** Your baby will be able to prop themselves up on their elbows, lift their head, and look around while they lie on their stomach.

- **Four months:** Your baby will begin to reach for and take hold of toys or other objects.

- **From 4 to 6 months:** Your baby will be able to roll from their back to their tummy and then roll back from their tummy onto their back.

- **From 5 to 6 months:** Your baby will be able to grab their feet with their hands while on their back and could start learning how to sit up while supported.

You can help encourage these advancements and further your child along the path of motor skill development. Shake rattle toys to get their interest and entice them to reach for them. Place toys in your child's hands to help them learn to grasp things. Lie on the floor beside them during tummy time and place items near their reach. Purchase hanging toys to place above them when they have floor-time play on their back so they can swipe at the objects. Play peek-a-boo, sing songs, and move colorful objects side-to-side to strengthen the baby's ability to follow things with their eyes.

In Summary

Welcoming a baby changes your life in many ways. You may need weeks or months to adjust to all the newness. In this chapter, we addressed many of these transitions, from bringing the baby home from the hospital to car safety, sleeping tips, and feeding options. We also checked in on your emotions and learned about some milestones you can expect your baby to achieve over their first six months.

As you begin your parenting journey, be kind to yourself. Let go of any pre-existing ideas you may have had about how things *should* be and embrace the daily joys and occasional challenges of your new family.

In the next chapter, we will discuss your baby's hygiene as well as their overall medical needs.

Chapter 3

Promoting Health and Well-Being

We have a secret in our culture, and it's not that birth is painful. It's that women are strong. —Laura Stavoe Harm

Newborns can be complicated beings, and while your flu symptoms as an adult may be quite straightforward to treat, a newborn cannot take medication—or even blow their noses for that matter.

Unfortunately, babies don't come with an instruction manual, but there are a couple of things you can learn upfront to have a smoother transition into the care and health of your newborn.

Bathing and Grooming

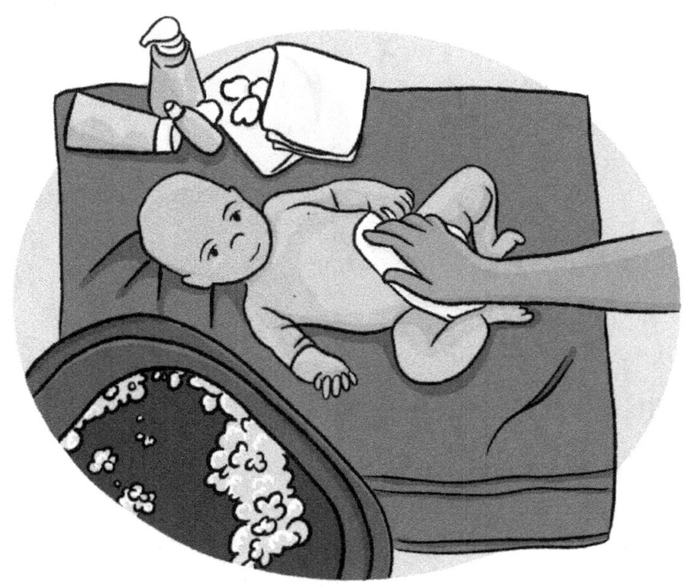

How Often to Bathe

The first bath that your baby will have will be very soon after delivery. Some parents like to have their babies bathed immediately, which has been a longstanding tradition, while some may give it a day or two as newer research has proven the benefits on the baby's skin if you wait (Carter, 2023).

Bathing can seem like a very daunting task to do with a newborn. They are so small and fragile, and water can be so dangerous. Fortunately, there are many tools and accessories that can help make bathing a baby a lot easier!

It is recommended that you bathe your newborn once or twice a week until their umbilical cord falls off. Try not to submerge them into the water entirely until this has happened to lower the risk of infection. At this time, you can use a washcloth to wipe them down in a sponge bath fashion. Once the cord has fallen off, you can bathe your newborn about three times a week, or less if you would like. Their skin is still very delicate, and frequent bathing may cause skin irritation or dryness. Newborns don't tend to get very dirty as they are pretty much sleeping all the time, so you do not need to worry about bathing them every day.

When bathing, start at the head and work your way down. Remember to let the warm water wash over their bellies as this will help ease any gas or tummy pains that they could be experiencing. Also, check all of their creases, especially in the neck area, and give it a good wipe to remove any dirt or milk residue.

If you see that your baby is having a reaction after a bath, then you may need to change their body wash to a fragrance-free brand.

At around three to six months, you can increase the baths to every second or third day if your baby enjoys the water, or if it forms part of your nighttime routine. Daily bathing is still not necessary at this stage, however.

Once your baby has started solids and is on the move, they will get dirty more frequently so you can bathe them as the need arises. You still do not need to bathe them every day, but you can increase the number of baths they have per week. You can also give them a sponge bath on the in between days.

Hair and Nail Care

Babies will often come straight out of the womb with long, sharp nails. This means that you will have to give their nails a trim a lot sooner than you would have liked! Cutting a tiny newborn's fingernails can be one of the most nerve-wracking tasks that you will ever have to perform.

From there, this task might become part of your weekly or bi-weekly routine. Babies' nails need to be kept very short as they can scratch themselves and others quite badly if their nails are even the littlest bit long. Fortunately, toenails grow at a less rapid rate and can, therefore, be cut about once a month.

Once you have gotten through the first trim or two, it will get easier. You should not harm your baby as long you remain focused and attentive.

How to Cut a Newborn's Nails

Here is a step-by-step guideline on how to effectively cut your newborn's nails:

1. Place your newborn on your lap in such a way that her head is snuggled into your chest and facing away from you.

2. Hold your baby's finger using your thumb and forefinger. Position the baby scissors or clippers gently under the nail.

3. Check to make sure that it is the nail and not skin that you are holding between the clippers. Initially, trim off tiny pieces only.

4. Once you are confident about trimming your newborn's nail, you can cut the entire nail at one go.

5. Cut toenails in a straight line and fingernails along the curve.

6. In case you are not confident about scissors or clippers for newborn nail care, make use of a smooth emery board.

7. Gently file down the rough pieces of the nail.

This process requires a little practice and a lot of patience. As you will be doing this routine on a weekly basis, you should start getting the hang of it in no time!

How to Care for Your Newborn's Hair

Your newborn's hair shouldn't be washed on a daily basis as it's very thin and delicate at this stage, so is the skin. Daily washing can cause the natural oils to be stripped and cradle cap can set in.

When it's time to wash your baby's hair, make sure that you use a gentle shampoo and that you rub your baby's scalp thoroughly and gently. As with the body wash, if you see any kind of reaction or a lot of cradle cap, then try using a different brand of shampoo or look for a natural alternative.

For the first few months, you should block your child's ears when rinsing their hair. Try to keep their ears as dry as possible throughout the bath time to avoid ear infections.

Once your baby's hair has been washed, dry it with a towel and use a soft bristle brush or comb to tidy it all up. You should avoid hair bands or any hairstyles that will pull too tightly on the scalp.

Diaper Rash

Diaper rashes can be quite common and happen when their diapers aren't changed frequently enough, or no preventative creams or solutions are applied. It is best to avoid diaper rashes and make use of the products that exist to keep the area dry and protected. It's only normal that a baby would be irritable and unsettled if they have a rash in the diaper area; I'm sure you can imagine what that would feel like, and it's not pleasant.

If your child does get a diaper rash, you can try rinsing your baby's bottom with warm water after each diaper change. Gently pat down the area with a towel to dry, or you can allow it to air dry for a couple of minutes (this may be the less painful method depending on the severity of the rash). You can then apply a cream, lotion, or ointment. In the past, mothers were told to use baby powder to keep the diaper area dry, however, this is no longer recommended as the powder has shown to have negative effects on the baby's lungs if inhaled (AAD, n.d.).

You should also keep an eye on the products that you are using, or even the brand of diapers as these could be causing the rash instead of preventing it.

Vaccinations and Medical Checkups

Vaccinations can be a bit of a controversial topic and every family may feel differently about them. However, the standard recommendation is that you immunize your baby as per the CDC's schedule (2019).

This schedule has been put together by healthcare professionals and considers the ideal time for your baby to receive the necessary vaccinations. The goal of vaccinations is for your baby's body to build an immunity against the virus that they receive. This will help your baby to fight off these ailments should they come into contact with them throughout their lives.

Choosing a Healthcare Provider

Many people are led to believe that they need to stick to the pediatrician who checked out their baby at the hospital after they were delivered. However, you are in total control of who you would like your child to see. You must make sure that you feel completely comfortable with the doctor and that their values are aligned with your own. You should decide what's important to you when it comes to your baby's health and the doctor you would like for them. It is also better to find someone in your area as you may need to call on them a couple of times throughout your child's life or in the event of an emergency.

If you are unsure, you can put together a list of questions to ask the pediatrician at your baby's first appointment. Doctors are accustomed to first-time parents, and they are usually quite accommodating in allaying your concerns.

Also, note that a pediatrician may not be necessary for every immunization. You can also find baby clinics or private nurses who administer these vaccinations.

Your pediatrician will be there to help with fevers, ear infections, and any other problems that you may encounter in your child's first few years.

Immunization Schedule

The standard schedule for immunizations for children based in the United States are as follows (CDC, 2019):

- **Birth:** First dose of Hepatitis B

- **One month:** Second dose of Hepatitis B

- **Two months:** DTaP, HiB, IPV, PVC, RV

The following months will be second and third doses of the vaccinations that were given at the two-month mark. Third doses of vaccinations may be required depending on what brand was given at the onset.

- **One year:** Measles, mumps, rubella, chickenpox, PVC

- **Two years:** Hepatitis A and DTap

- **Six years:** DTAP, MMR, IPV and Varicella

There are also a couple of vaccinations that your child will be required to get during their teenage years.

Illness

It can be very difficult to tell if your baby is sick simply because they are unable to communicate yet. Where a toddler can tell you that their tummy aches or their ears hurt, babies only know one way of talking to you: crying. However, crying is also what they use to tell you that they are hungry, tired, or just bored. So, how do you know when something is seriously wrong?

Your first hint should be that your baby is not only crying, but they are crying or groaning constantly. You should then check for a fever, which is a common telltale sign that your baby's body is experiencing something severe. The following can also be looked out for:

- vomiting or diarrhea

- lethargy

- infection of any kind (check ears, umbilical cord)

- loss of appetite

If your baby is experiencing one or more of the following, there's a good chance that they are sick. There's not much in the way of medication available for babies under the age of three months; however, you can ask your local pharmacist for advice and recommendations before driving to the pediatrician.

Emergencies

If your baby is showing signs of any of the following, then head straight to the emergency room:

- your baby can't wake up, is not moving, or is very weak.

- they are making moaning or grunting noises while breathing.

- their lips, tongue, or face have a blue or gray tinge.

- severe coughing, diarrhea, or vomiting

- severe sweating

- struggling to feed

- the soft spot on their head is sunken or swollen.

- sleeping much more than normal

- Your baby is younger than 12 weeks old and has a fever.

- Their temperature is below 96.8°F and does not increase with warming up.

- Their temperature is over 104°F and does not cool down.

Along with these tell-tale signs, it is also important to rely on your gut. As the mother, or guardian of the child, you will know when something is wrong with them. It is better to take them to the doctor or emergency room and be sent home than to ignore it and they become seriously harmed.

Soothing and Comforting Baby

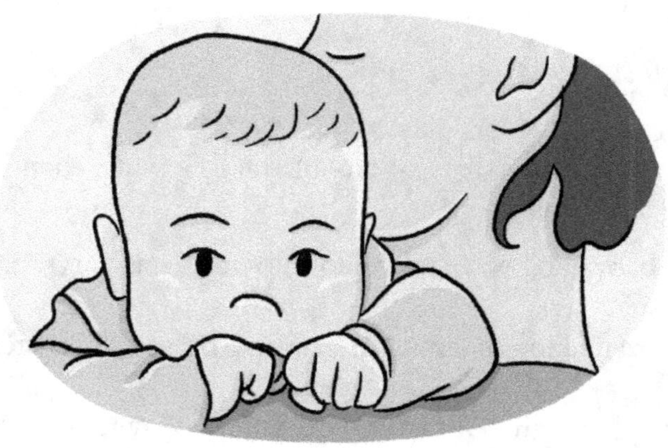

There will be many instances in your newborn's life where you will need to sooth or comfort them. Babies are unable to take a hold of their emotions, so any discomfort or surge of emotions that they feel, they will make known to you! Each baby might have different methods of comfort and soothing that they prefer. Some might take a pacifier, others might like to be sung to. But, in some instances, common techniques and practices can make the difference.

Colic and Gas

If you are breastfeeding and your baby has frequent colic or gas problems, it might be wise to take a look at your diet. Keep a food journal over a period of two weeks and track your baby's mood with each day. You may find that on the days that you have that extra cup of coffee, your baby tends to experience some discomfort. Newborns are very sensitive to the foods that breastfeeding moms consume. Some foods that cause gas in babies include broccoli, caffeine, cauliflower, onion, and sometimes even dairy products.

If you are unsure which food could be causing their tummy troubles, then try to eliminate one food for a period of two weeks and see whether that could be the one. This may seem like a tedious and drawn-out process, but it does take a while for traces of the food to completely work its way out of your baby's system. Hopefully you will find the correct food on the first try!

For bottle-fed babies, try swapping the brand of formula that you are using. You can consult your family's healthcare provider for recommendations based on your baby's specific needs and symptoms.

Burping is also a key part to relieving discomfort from newborns. This may take some time and practice to ace, but it will be well worth the effort. You can also try feeding your baby smaller quantities more frequently in order to alleviate some pressure off of their digestive system.

If you've tried everything and your baby is just colicky, and the crying and discomfort continue, try investing in a good carrier so that you can carry your baby around on your body while you continue with what you need to get done for the day. Babies tend to be calmer and more relaxed the closer they are to you, as the warmth from your body soothes them and helps them settle down.

Baby Exercises and Massage

Massages and exercises are so important for your baby's development and it's also a great way to relieve any tension that's in their bodies.

Tummy time is one of the most recommended activities that you can do with your baby. Healthcare professionals recommend doing at least 15 minutes of tummy time, a few times throughout the day (Cleveland Clinic, 2022b). Tummy time will help strengthen their neck, back, and arms muscles, which then leads to bigger milestones such as holding up their heads independently and crawling.

Babies who have tummy cramps can benefit greatly from tummy time as this will help release any stuck gas and it will be a soothing process. Remember to always make sure that tummy time is a supervised activity.

Massaging your baby can equally help relieve any aches and pains that they are feeling and is a great way to get them to relax. Massaging them after a bath is a good time, as their muscles will be warmed up and, therefore, more supple.

Rub their tummies in circular motions, do bicycles with their legs, and rub the soles of their feet. Start at the head and work your way down, making sure to spend a minute or two on each section of the body.

Teething

If any of your friends or family members are parents to small children, you would've most likely heard about the horrors of teething! Don't panic though, as it's not always as bad as people make it out to be.

Teething is the process in which the baby's teeth cut through the gums and grow. Yes, it is as painful as it sounds, especially for a tiny baby who doesn't even know what a tooth is. As much as you may be desperate for a good night's sleep, remember that it's your baby who is ultimately going through the painful process and is crying out for you to help them through it.

When your baby is teething, pain medication, as well as refrigerated chewy toys, will be the go-to remedies. Check your baby for any signs of a fever as this is a common teething symptom.

In Summary

Newborn healthcare can be complicated as you don't always know what's wrong with your baby or what to do about it. A simple and mild fever can quickly escalate, and you will find yourself rushing to the ER. The main thing to remember is to remain as prepared as possible and to follow the guidelines given throughout this chapter. If you are unsure, your best bet is to go see a doctor or go straight to the hospital. Medical staff are used to new parents and would rather that you take the extra precaution than leave it and a more serious condition arise.

In the next chapter, we will go through the benefits of attending to your child's needs and cries in order to develop a deep bond and the development benefits thereof.

Chapter 4:

Emotional Development and Family Bonding

That first pregnancy is a long sea journey to a country where you don't know the language, where land is in sight for such a long time that after a while it's just the horizon—and then, one day, birds wheel over that dark shape and it's suddenly close, and all you can do is hope like hell that you've had the right shots. —Emily Perkins

Bonding with your baby is every parent or caregiver's dream. Would all of it be worth it if a positive bond didn't form after months of care and nurturing? You will find that over time, your baby will be very reliant and in need of you, and you will also need them and rely on their presence and overall happiness.

It is only natural that your baby will cling to their primary caregiver and this stems back to their survival instinct. The person that feeds them, will be the person that they never want to lose sight of. This is especially evident in the first couple of months before the baby's social skills set in. Babies will go through periods where they will be completely attached to their mothers and will even experience separation anxiety if she is not around.

Responding to Baby's Needs

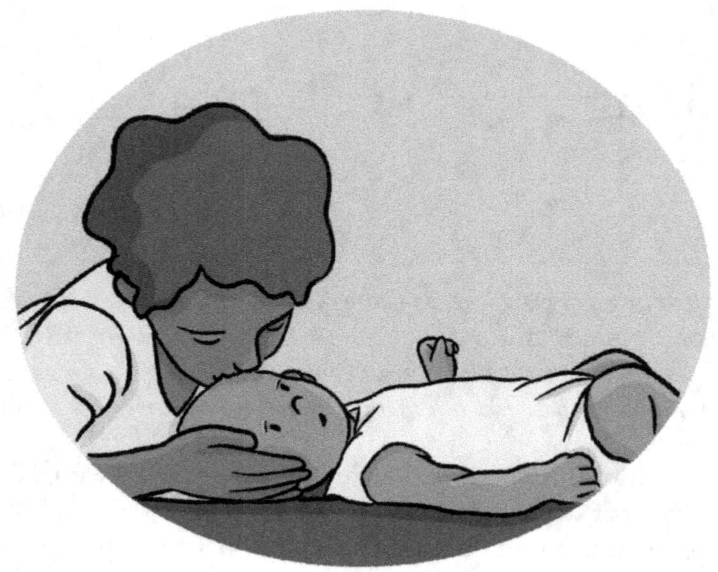

Being responsive to your baby's needs is a very important part of parenthood. This not only helps to make your baby feel secure and loved, but it also gives them the confidence boost that they need to reach their developmental milestones. Research has shown some of the benefits of children who have a good relationship with their parents in early childhood include better problem-solving skills and higher academic achievements. On the contrary, babies who feel neglected will have lifelong effects on their development and character formation (FHS, 2018).

Why Responsive Care Is Important

The term "responsive care" is as simple as it sounds. This basically means that you are caring for your baby by responding to what they need. By paying attention and providing your child with what they need or want when they ask for it, you are showing them that they matter to you. This does not mean that you have to buy your child every toy that they want for years to come. This is specifically referring to the early childhood years and mainly consists of essential care such as food, physical touch, nurturing, and so on.

By responding to your baby's call, you are encouraging them to communicate with you. If your child's cries fall on deaf ears, they will eventually stop trying to communicate, which will lead to language and speech difficulties later on down the line. It will also cause trust issues as the baby will feel that there is no one to care for them or attend to their needs. They are basically on their own. No matter how small your baby is, it's important that you recognize when they need you and try your best to sort them out as soon as you can. Some signs to look out for—depending on the child's age—include rubbing their eyes to signal tiredness, pointing, or crying to signal discomfort or hunger.

Baby Wearing

Baby wearing is when you carry or "wear" your baby on your body using a carrier, wrap, or sling. You can carry baby facing inward (with their face toward your chest) which is an ideal position for newborns, outward (face turning away from you), or on your back.

When wearing your baby, they feel more secure and at ease. This is a great way to settle them while you are continuing to get stuff done around the house, or even out running errands. If you have ever traveled to Africa, you will notice that the majority of the women go about their daily work or errands with their babies tied to their back using a simple blanket or towel. You will also notice that these babies are very content, are not crying, and are simply happy being close to their moms while she gets her work done. The mom will also be at ease and happy knowing that her baby is safe and comfortable, and she has her hands free in order to get her tasks done.

If your baby tends to cry a lot and you feel like they can never be put down without a fight, then you may want to consider purchasing a carrier. It has been proven to reduce crying, and can include even up to 51% reduced crying in the evening time (Marcin, 2019). Some other benefits may include bonding, better success at breastfeeding, and positive growth for the baby.

However, it is vital that you are carrying your baby safely! If done incorrectly, or with the wrong type of carrier, it can do more harm than good for your child. Practitioners and parents refer to the T.I.C.K.S method to determine whether your baby is safe in their carrier. These refer to "T" (Tight), "I" (In View), "C" (Close), "K" (Keep Chin Off Chest), and "S" (Supported Back (and neck for newborns)).

If you want to start wearing your baby from birth, then make sure that your carrier is supportive enough for a newborn's neck.

Promoting Emotional Milestones

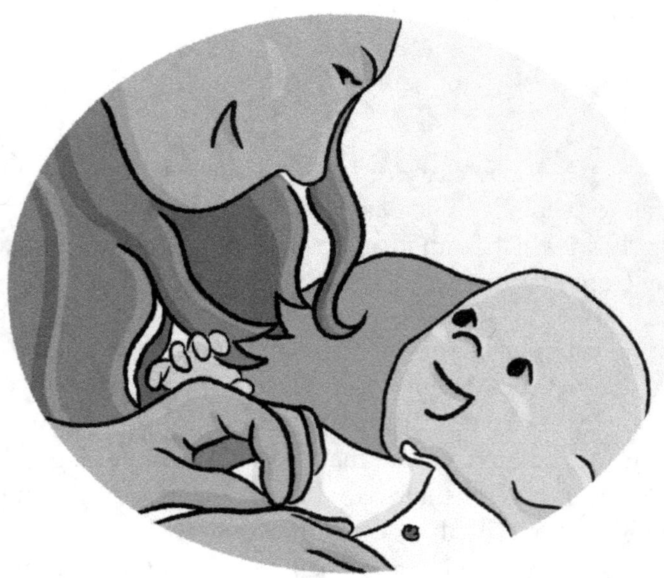

Many parents focus on physical milestones such as sitting, crawling, and walking. However, there are a lot of social and emotional milestones that a baby needs to work toward and achieve. Social skills are vital in this day and age as we live in a time where communicating with others is a vital skill. Although it may seem like children only learn social skills when they start school, this is actually not the case. A child learns to socially interact when they are a baby.

Social Interactions

A significant part of your baby's brain development is geared toward studying, remembering, and recognizing faces, as well as facial expressions. You may think that it's pointless to talk to a five-month-old because they don't even understand what you are saying, but they are learning so much just by watching your face and the expressions you are making. The tone of your voice will also be picked up on and your baby will very quickly be able to distinguish which tone is loving and which is anger.

You may find around the six-month mark that your baby will giggle when you do a sudden expression such as shock or surprise. As adults, when we get to know someone on a personal level, we tend to make a lot of eye contact and observe how that person talks. It's no different with a baby. They are making connections with the people around them every single day and are forming a strong tie to their immediate family members. They want you to talk to them, look them in the eyes, make them laugh, surprise them, and spend time connecting.

If you feel awkward talking to your baby, then try singing to them. You can then move toward describing things like sounds or things that they are seeing. For example, if you are out for a walk and a dog barks, you can say "doggy, woof woof." Even the smallest of interactions will be beneficial for your baby.

Social Milestones

There are a couple of key milestones to look out when it comes to your baby's social milestones which are:

- first smile (around two to three months old)

- change in cries depending on their needs (around three months)

- recognizing their name (between three and six months)

- reaching arms out to you (around six months)

- babbling and saying first words (around six months)

- pointing (between six to twelve months)

- separation anxiety (between six to twelve months)

Naturally, the older your baby gets, the more milestones they will reach such as talking, teasing, and singing.

Do not be alarmed if some of the milestones may seem negative, like separation anxiety. As adults, this has a very negative connotation to it, but it is a crucial part to a baby's development as it usually happens when they start learning more about themselves as an individual being.

Positive Interactions

In the early years, it is extremely beneficial for your child if you keep interactions as positive as possible. The primary years will mold and shape your child into who they will become in the future.

If your child is led to believe that interactions with their parents or caregivers results in a negative experience, they will tend to retreat and become very anti-social. They will not see the point in needing to communicate if every interaction seems to lead to trouble. For this reason, try to keep your daily communication with your baby light-hearted, loving, and positive.

Playing with your child is a great way to help them enjoy interacting with others and it will allow them the confidence that they need to reach out. Reading can also form part of positive interaction and social activities. You should also try to limit the number of times that you use negative words on a daily basis such as "no." When your child is trying to communicate with you, make sure that you are attentive and make eye contact whenever possible.

Self-Soothing and Independence

Another key milestone for babies is learning to self-soothe. Self-soothing is, essentially, the baby learning to put themselves to sleep (or back to sleep) with minimal crying. They are learning to be more independent, to be calm, and to reassure themselves without needing a parent or caregiver to intervene. The reason why parents encourage and train their babies to self-soothe is to relieve pressure off of themselves by having to wake up multiple times a night to attend to the baby, which could lead to extreme fatigue, burnout, and depression.

Between the ages of three and six months, babies should start experiencing a more stabilized sleeping pattern and many will be sleeping through the night by six months. However, it is also not uncommon for a baby to still be waking frequently for the first year. This can often be due to a sleep-crutch that the baby has developed, such as comfort feeding and rocking. By teaching your child to self-soothe, you are eliminating those crutches, which will result in a better night's sleep all around.

To set yourself (and your little one) up for success, have a routine in place so your baby knows when and where they are expected to sleep. Make sure that their environment is as peaceful as possible (use blackout curtains, white noise, and temperature control). Avoid nursing, rocking, or swaying your baby to sleep. Instead, lay them in their crib and leave them for a little while to soothe themselves.

You must start gradually (with a couple of minutes) and slowly work your way up. Two minutes may sound like a short amount of time, but it can be very long if your baby is crying nonstop. Remain close to the baby's room so that you can monitor their crying and go to them if you hear that they are going into distress.

Preparing Siblings for the Arrival of a Newborn

Older siblings can have a hard time processing the thought of a newer member of the family. Depending on their age, they may be excited the first few hours, but they will soon realize that their whole world has been turned upside down. They are no longer the center of attention, or the only child who needs you.

They will have to make big changes to fit into the family and their relationship with you will suddenly change. They will have to become more independent overnight. Where they would usually have positive interactions with you, they will now be told constantly "Keep it down, the baby is sleeping," "Be gentle with the baby," or "Mommy can't help you right now. I am feeding the baby." These can all feel like harsh words to a child who just wants things to go back to how they were.

You may feel overwhelmed with the new addition yourself but remember that your little one doesn't have as much control over their emotions as you do. They also cannot process what is happening as well as an adult. It's a time when communication—especially the positive kind—will be essential.

Young children (between the ages of one and two) will not entirely understand the concept of a sibling and what that means. The goal will then be to get them as excited as possible. They will learn to be happy and excited for the arrival of their sibling when your excitement rubs off on them.

Make sure to talk about baby brother or sister very often and let them help you set up the nursery, pick out the baby clothes, and get the home ready for the new arrival. You can also read lots of books to them about siblings and babies. The shock of a new baby will still be evident though once the sibling is brought into the house, so make sure to give your older child lots of attention and love in order to reassure them during the transition period.

Older children (between the ages of two and four) may understand more than the previous age group, but they will still need to be eased into the process. At this age, you will be able to communicate a lot more and explain to your older child what having a sibling entails such as crying, sharing attention, and that the baby won't do much for the first couple of months.

Children who are older than five years of age will be much easier to prepare than the previous age groups. They will not see a new baby as a threat, but rather as a reason to be excited. At this age, they will be a lot more interested in playing with friends or toys than sitting with mommy all day, so they won't be desperate for your attention. School and activities will also take their mind off of things; however, you still need to make sure that your older child doesn't feel pushed aside or neglected because of the baby. A good way to get them involved is to give them some baby-related tasks, or a part of the baby care that will be theirs to do such as putting cream on the baby or choosing their outfits for the day.

Pets

While introducing a new pet to the family is, by no means, as intricate or stressful as introducing a new baby, it can still feel overwhelming for a small child.

The main goal in this instance is to ensure that everyone remains safe and at ease throughout the process. Your baby may want to constantly be around your pet, touching them, pulling their tails, and remaining in their space constantly; but, remember that your pet will also need some time to adjust and, depending on the animal, they may have a negative reaction to an action that they don't like (such as a pull of the tail).

To keep everyone in control, make sure that you are present whenever your child and pet interact over the first couple of weeks. You will then be able to gauge where the boundaries need to be set in order to ensure everyone's safety. It is also good to keep an eye on whether your baby has allergy symptoms toward your pet's hair. These can include skin irritation (such as hives or welts), watery eyes, sneezing, and wheezing.

Other Family Members

When relying on extended family members to help look after or care for your child, there is some tactfulness required. Boundaries can easily be stepped over when a family member is close to the child, yet not the child's actual parent, is babysitting.

In a first instance, you can overstep a boundary by asking your family to babysit very frequently and with no pay. While you don't have to give them cold, hard cash, buying their meal for the day or giving some money for gas and an outing is always appreciated. Unless the family member explicitly says so, it should not be assumed that they will constantly be looking after your child at their own expense—especially if it could put them in an uncomfortable financial situation. Try to see it as a way of saying "thank you" to them for taking the time to look after your child.

It is also important that you make rules and regulations very clear to anyone who looks after your child. Things like discipline, expectations, and specifics relating to your child should be discussed and agreed upon in advance.

In Summary

There is more to your baby than just crawling, rolling, and walking. They are little human beings, which means that they have a wide array of emotions, thoughts, needs, and feelings. All of these need to be taken care of and attended to in order for your baby to grow up feeling confident and loved.

Throughout the next chapter, we will explore the importance of play and how this can help your child throughout their lives.

Chapter 5:

Cognitive and Motor Development

Children learn as they play. Most importantly, in play, children learn how to learn.
—O. Fred Donaldson

You have probably heard the saying that a baby is like a sponge. It is so easy for them to absorb information and learn new things. Studies have shown that one of the hardest things for an adult to do is learn a new language. However, toddlers and young children can learn multiple languages quite easily (Arnon, 2023). Because they have a clean slate, they can quickly grasp new concepts, unlike adults who have a lot of stored habits, ideas, and mannerisms that make it harder for them to conform to anything new. Let's face it, if your mouth has been used to moving the same way for over 20 years, it will take some time for it to learn new movements and sounds.

Stimulation and Early-Learning: Age-Appropriate Toys and Activities

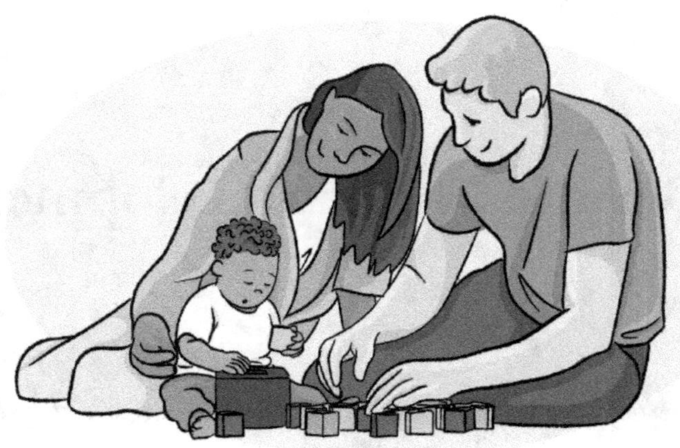

Playtime and toys are an excellent way to get your little one to learn and be stimulated healthily. The types of toys that you choose will make a great impact on what they learn going forward. For example, toys that are hard plastic and don't do anything but shine bright lights and play loud, fast tunes will prove to be of little benefit to your child's development.

By buying toys that are useful and practical for day-to-day activities, you are allowing your little one to develop their abilities in a positive and constructive manner.

Activities

Young Infants (First Six Months)

In the first six months of life, children will need toys that make noise, are easy to reach for and hold, textured, teething-friendly, and able to be put in the mouth safely. Simple music is a must at this age in order to avoid overstimulating the baby and keep them in a calm and secure environment.

They may not be into books or anything visual at this stage; however, you could try getting a baby-friendly handheld mirror as they will be taking an interest in studying their faces at this age.

Older Infants (Seven Months to One Year)

The toys will start getting more complicated from this point on. By now, your baby will probably be crawling and getting ready to walk, so moveable toys with wheels or balls would be a good idea at this stage to encourage movement.

Repetition and problem-solving will also start to surface. Activities and toys that they need to stack, pack, organize, or resolve will be a great hit! Your baby might also start taking an interest in soft dolls and stuffed animals.

Beyond One Year

Drawing, singing, and imaginary play will be a general go-to at this age. While this is still the beginning stage, you can buy your child toys and activities in line with these, and you will notice that they will play with these items more and more.

Your child will also be going through an independent phase and will want to do as much as possible on their own. This will be a good time to get them involved in chores around the house. Let them help you with cooking, cleaning, tidying up, and caring for other members of the household. Bear in mind that having little hands help you might take longer and feel unproductive in getting things done, but this is such a great way for them to learn and be with you at the same time.

No matter the age group, remember to include all of the baby's senses in their playing experience. Different shapes, colors, sizes, materials, and sounds can be beneficial to helping them enhance their sensory experience through play.

Tummy Time and Motor Skills

If you're a new parent, you have most likely heard the words "tummy time" hundreds of times. Great emphasis is often placed on the need to have your child do tummy time and all the benefits that come with this. The only challenge is that most babies are not fond of tummy time. At least, they do not enjoy being on their tummies for as long as the recommended times. Do not feel discouraged, however. Every baby is different, and any amount of tummy time is better than none at all.

The term "tummy time" is quite self-explanatory, but for the sake of reference, it means to lay a baby on their tummy. This should generally be on a flat, even surface; and is something that many doctors, childcare professionals, and other parents would highly recommend doing daily, starting with a couple of minutes and working your way up. Being on their tummies is a great way for them to strengthen muscles that will be essential to reaching certain milestones, such as holding up their heads without support, rolling, and even crawling. Babies who don't do tummy time as much will still reach these milestones, however, it will most likely be at a much slower pace than the tummy time enthusiasts.

You can start tummy time with your newborn as soon as they are home from the hospital. Don't expect much in the first few weeks, but eventually, you will see your baby lifting their head more and more. If your baby isn't enjoying lying on their tummies, you can try dangling a toy or an interesting object in front of them. This is a great time to start bonding with your newborn and figuring out their likes and dislikes.

During tummy time, it's important that you stay in the room and watch over your child. While it is a fairly safe exercise, there are still risks to it so it's best to keep an eye out at all times. The main thing you want to look for is that their face (especially the mouth and nose) is not directly against the ground as this will prevent your baby from breathing. It is also good to remember that tummy time is an activity that must be done when your baby is awake. Your baby should not be asleep while on their tummies.

Exercises

There are several exercises that will help your baby strengthen their muscles as well as promote coordination during the first year of life. These include:

- rolling

- pull into a sitting position (*Note:* Pull from shoulders and not from wrist to avoid dislocating the arm)

- sitting in between your legs and playing with toys on the ground

- creeping

- crawling

- kneeling

- sit to stand

- weight-shifting

- step up

You can do all of these exercises with your baby, at the right age, before they can do these independently. Make sure that you give them lots of physical support and that you help them in a way that they will learn the pattern and be able to do the same things independently. Decrease the amount of support and guidance that you give to them by a little bit every day and they will soon learn to take over.

Tracking Developmental Milestones

Observing and tracking milestones is an important part of the parental journey as it lets you know whether your baby is achieving all that they should be for their age, and it helps you as well as your healthcare provider pick up on whether there could be any developmental problems with your child at an early stage.

Unfortunately, milestone tracking can prove to be a stressful process for new parents as they will feel under pressure to have their baby perform when they should, or even earlier than the norm. This can especially be the case in big families or friend groups where there are multiple babies. However, it's important to remember that every baby is different, and putting pressure on yourself and your baby to reach milestones is not constructive.

When you went to high school did anyone ask you what month you started crawling? Or during your first job interview, did they want to know how old you were when you took your first few steps? In the grand scheme of life, baby milestones are not a big deal. That being said, it's important that you track them and report back to your healthcare provider if you think that there is a cause for concern.

Milestones are divided into four categories: motor, sensory, feeding, and communication. These categories will cover all the bases of your child's development and what they should know at each stage.

Motor Milestones

Motor milestones include:

- brings hands to mouth (zero to three months)

- moves body, kicks, and moves arms when excited (zero to three months)

- rolls from back to tummy and vice versa (four to six months)

- stands with entire weight on legs with the support of an adult (four to six months)

- reaches for toys (four to six months)

- plays with or grabs feet while lying on back (four to six months)

- sits unsupported (seven to nine months)

- moves from a lying position to a sitting position (seven to nine months)

- starts making creeping or crawling movements (seven to nine months)

- tracks items with eyes and movement of the head (seven to nine months)

- pulls themselves up in a standing position (ten to twelve months)

- cruises along furniture (ten to twelve months)

- claps (ten to twelve months)

- able to pick up small objects (ten to twelve months)

Sensory Milestones

Sensory milestones include:

- tries to reach for dangling toys while they are lying down (zero to three months)

- visually tracks big items (zero to three months)

- is soothed by rocking or swaying (zero to three months)

- uses both hands to touch and hold toys (four to six months)

- overall content attitude unless hungry or tired (four to six months)

- used to everyday sounds (four to six months)

- enjoys lots of different types of movement (seven to nine months)

- observes and examines objects shapes, sizes, and textures (seven to nine months)

- looks around at surroundings (seven to nine months)

- listens to music (ten to twelve months)

- crawls to objects that can be seen from afar (ten to twelve months)

Communication Milestones

Communication milestones include:

- keeps quiet when hearing your voice (zero to three months)

- begins to smile (zero to three months)

- makes eye contact (zero to three months)

- cries change depending on need (zero to three months)

- reacts to sudden noise (four to six months)

- starts babbling (four to six months)

- enjoys toys with sound and music (four to six months)

- may start calling out for your attention (four to six months)

- can recognize people's names (seven to nine months)

- tries to hold a conversation (seven to nine months)

- increased babbling (seven to nine months)

- can follow gestures and commands (seven to nine months)

- calls for "mama" or "dada" (ten to twelve months)

- imitates sounds and noises (ten to twelve months)

- knows one or two words (ten to twelve months)

- understands and responds to certain words like "no" or "where?" (ten to twelve months)

Feeding Milestones

Feeding milestones include:

- latches onto breast or bottle (zero to three months)

- swallows (zero to three months)

- looks at food and shows interest (four to six months)

- starts solids such as porridge and purees (four to six months)

- can have meals in a designated chair (seven to nine months)

- solids become more textured (seven to nine months)

- can self-feed using fingers (ten to twelve months)

- use of an open cup (ten to twelve months)

- wide range of food (ten to twelve months)

Developmental Delays

Some of the problems to watch out for are mainly related to your baby's sight, hearing, speech, body strength, and temperament. If you notice anything odd or peculiar then speak to your healthcare provider as soon as possible.

If there are indeed developmental delays, as confirmed by your healthcare provider, then try to get to a specialist quickly to see whether anything can be done through early intervention. You will need to provide lots of love, care, patience, and support to your child as they won't understand what is going on. Remember that through all of this, you are their safe space. You may have moments of frustration, which is completely normal. During these times, make sure that there is someone around who can help you look after your child so that you can get out and clear your mind a bit.

In Summary

As Vivienne Borne from Maryland said "Nothing else can produce the joy or broken heart that motherhood allows. I couldn't imagine going through life without feeling that spectrum of emotion. There are wonderful days when I feel my cup runneth over. There are days that I want to run away and question every decision I have ever made. Feeling it all, good or bad, gives my life purpose. Motherhood is walking around with all of your nerve endings raw and exposed. It is the most extreme measure of being alive."

That is exactly the sentiment that most parents feel. Every journey is different but it is important that you do your best to track your baby's development and that you help and support them along the way. There are many resources available online or in bookstores and baby shops that can make tracking practical and fun. If in doubt, speak to a nurse or doctor who will then either be able to allay your concerns or refer you for further specialist intervention.

In the next chapter, we will touch on one of the most important aspects of childcare: sleep. Sleep methods and training are vital to how you cope as a new parent and can drastically affect your ability to function if it is lacking.

Chapter 6:

Sleep Solutions and Establishing Healthy Habits

Watching a baby sleep peacefully is perhaps the only thing more comfortable than sleep itself. —Anonymous

Newborns sleep a lot, just not all at once, which means you don't get a good quality sleep at all. Adults need at least seven hours of sleep per night. Tricia Youngblood of Sleepme says that during their baby's first year, moms lose about 90 minutes of sleep each night (2023). Take an hour and a half out of your seven every night of the year, and your mind and body will start to feel the consequences, like brain fog, fatigue, irritability, anxiety or depression, and potential long-term health effects.

According to AJ Hopper, author of *Find Your Mantra, Momma* (2023), being sleep-deprived can have the same effect on you as being drunk. Studies from the National Institute of Occupational Safety and Health have shown that going 17 hours without sleep causes similar cognitive and physiological impairment as having a blood content (BAC) of 0.05%, and not sleeping for 24 hours is equivalent to a BAC of 0.10%. To note, a BAC of 0.08% classifies someone as legally intoxicated in the United States. At just 0.05% BAC, effects are noticeable in a person's driving abilities (CDC, 2020).

Babies also need a lot of sleep to help them grow and be healthy too. Below is a list from WebMD showing how much sleep your baby needs at each stage of infancy (WebMD, 2022):

- **The first four weeks:** Newborns should sleep 15–16 hours—and up to 18 hours—every day. Preemies tend to sleep more, and colicky babies sleep less. However, most newborns don't sleep more than two to four hours at a time and have no regular sleep pattern.

- **One to four months:** The sleep requirement drops to 14–15 hours at this stage, and infants may sleep about four to six hours at a time. Soon, they will be attentive to day-night cycles, as their circadian rhythm develops.

- **Four to twelve months:** Ideally, babies still need about 14–15 hours of sleep per night at this stage, but some may sleep as little as 12 hours per day. Naps will also drop from three to two per day after about six months of age, and they should be able to sleep through the night.

As we progress through this chapter, we'll talk about sleep solutions you can easily implement for your baby *and* yourself.

Nurturing Healthy Sleep Habits

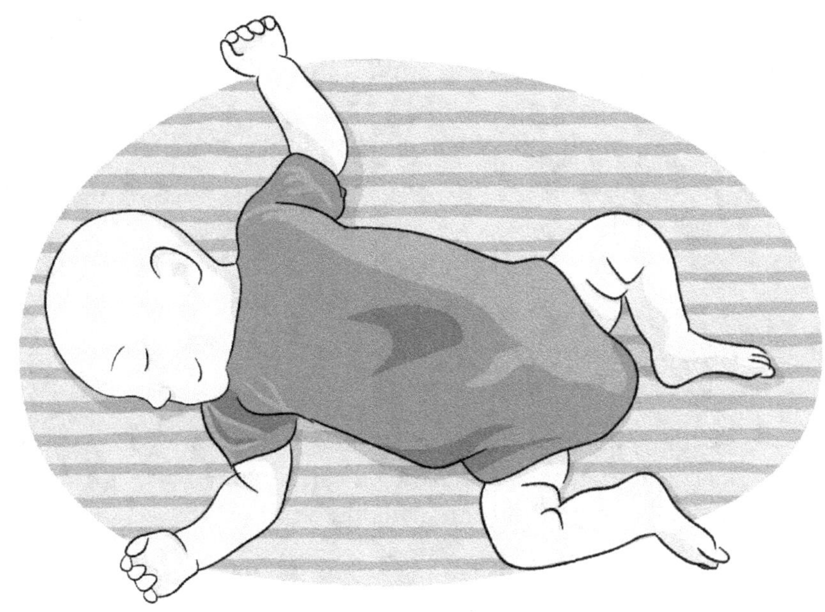

A large amount of the time newborns sleep in light sleep known as rapid eye movement (REM). Growth hormones are released during this light sleep, aiding in the child's development. Brain activity is also stimulated as cognitive development processes input it has received throughout the day. REM sleep also contributes to survival instincts, allowing the baby to awaken if they need more sustenance or if they are alerted to what they perceive to be a threat or danger. Some other reasons babies awake during the night are that their circadian rhythm hasn't developed, so they don't know if it's night or day; they're overexcited from too much stimulation; they are in pain or are ill; or they just simply need you.

Although your baby sleeps lightly and may awaken frequently, you should not immediately rush to console them. Unless they are hungry, wet, or in danger, they will likely fall back asleep on their own. Below are some other reasons to pause, listen, and assess before picking them up:

- Sometimes, like you, they just need to wiggle and stretch.

- If you immediately pick them up, they will form a habit of waking regularly so that you will come to them, and this will keep their sleep disrupted. They may also become reliant on your rocking, cuddling, or nursing for them to get back to sleep.

- Allowing them to go back to sleep on their own—assuming there is no real need to pick them up or soothe them—will help them cultivate sleep independence and self-regulation.

- They may simply be between sleep cycles, and if you pick them up, you will disrupt that and make it more difficult for them to fall back to sleep.

Sleep Training Your Infant

There are several approaches to managing a baby's sleep. A popular option is sleep training, which can begin when your baby is four to six months old. The basic methods are listed here:

- **Crying it out:** This method is just as it sounds, placing your baby in their bed and letting them cry until they fall asleep. Although it can take some infants hours to stop crying and go to sleep, proponents say this helps the child to become an independent sleeper who doesn't rely on Mom or Dad to soothe them.

- **Camping out:** In this method, you also allow your child to cry it out, but you remain in the room with them until they settle down. In theory, just your presence comforts them. Over time, the parent's time spent in the room is reduced until the infant can go to sleep independently.

- **Ferber method:** Again, similar to the cry-it-out method, you allow your child to cry when they're put to bed, but you check on them every 5, 10, or 15 minutes and pat their back, rub their head, or whisper or sing softly to soothe them. Extend the time interval each night.

- **Bedtime fading:** This is a no-cry method. You begin by putting your child to bed at a late time, like 10:00 p.m. It needs to be late enough that they feel the urge to sleep. Over the following days, you reduce the bedtime by 15 minutes until your child is falling asleep at your preferred time.

- **No tears:** This is a more gradual way to sleep train. You offer immediate comfort whenever your baby cries. You should assess the situation first, though, by following the tips we mentioned earlier.

"The 5 S's" are a tear-free, compassionate way to soothe your baby and help them sleep well. Let's take a look at what they are (Karp, n.d.):

1. **The 1st S:** Swaddle

2. **The 2nd S:** Side or Stomach Position

3. **The 3rd S:** Shush

4. **The 4th S:** Swing

5. **The 5th S:** Suck

By remembering these five S's you will be able to quickly settle your baby in a nurturing and comforting way.

Strategies for Managing Your Sleep Challenges

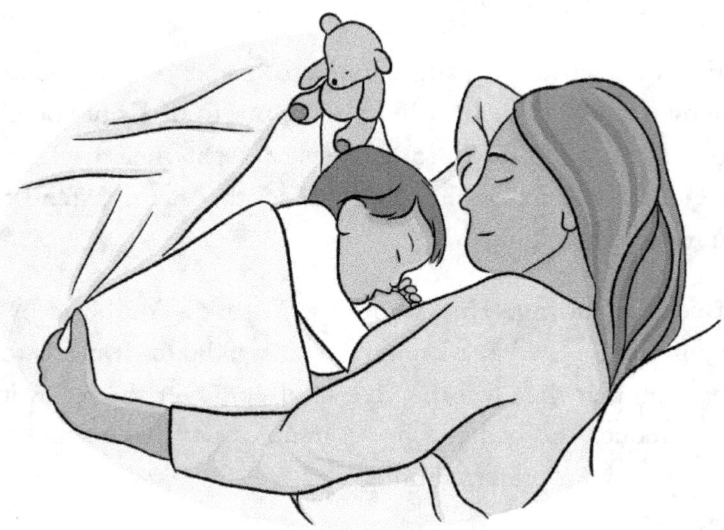

Helping your baby sleep better will give you the chance to improve your rest as well. You need adequate sleep to give your child your full attention, effectively tend to their needs and the needs of your family, and stay in prime health.

In addition, the National Heart, Lung, and Blood Institute (2022) says that "After several nights of losing sleep—even a loss of just one to two hours per night—your ability to function suffers as if you haven't slept at all for a day or two." Getting adequate sleep will give you more mental clarity, reduce irritability, decrease the risk of developing anxiety or depression, and improve long-term health effects.

Check out the following tips to keep your sleep sound and restorative:

- **Sleep when the baby sleeps:** This is probably the most common piece of advice people will give you, and it's probably the wisest too. Even if you're applying the tips we mentioned in the last section, it will still take your newborn time to adjust to life outside the womb—and that includes when to sleep and when not to. Your body has been through a lot of stress during pregnancy and childbirth, and now that you're adjusting to new responsibilities, you need all the rest you can get. Take advantage of the baby's downtime to give yourself some downtime too.

- **Avoid co-sleeping:** It's tempting to let the baby sleep in the bed with you, but that can be dangerous because you and your spouse may be restless sleepers and accidentally harm the baby without realizing it. Bedside cribs that sidle up to your bed are ideal for keeping the baby close to you. It will help you to relax and have a more peaceful sleep, knowing the baby is safe in their own space.

- **Limit sleep aids and energy boosts:** These supplements might help on occasion, but they can quickly become addictive and can affect your cognitive abilities. If you are breastfeeding, some of the components may pass through your milk to your baby and potentially harm them as well. Always consult your doctor if you feel the need for medical sleep assistance.

- **Eat a healthy diet and maintain some form of exercise:** "Eat the rainbow," incorporate lots of nutritious foods into every meal, and do some sort of physical activity for at least 30 minutes, 5 days a week.

- **Don't worry about a messy house:** The laundry will get done eventually. Your husband can cook the evening meal. Dishes and pans can wait until morning. When you need rest, put your household chores aside temporarily.

- **Ask for and accept help:** You don't have to be a super-parent and do everything yourself. It's okay to need a break. Have your spouse or partner take an overnight shift. Invite a grandparent over for an afternoon and let them tend to the baby while you take a nap. Take your friend up on their offer to babysit now and then.

- **Turn down invitations:** It's important to maintain your friendships and other acquaintances, but you don't have to attend every event you're invited to. People will understand that you may not have the mental or physical energy for it yet, so don't feel pressured to go everywhere you're called to go.

- **Don't rush sleep:** You may be tempted to rush to bed and try to fall asleep fast to get in as much rest as possible before the baby wakes up. That's not how your body works, though. Allow yourself time to unwind. Shut off electronic devices, televisions, and other things that may keep your mind active. Keep a cool temperature in your room, keep it dark and quiet, and let your mind and body settle in on their own time.

Strategies to Help Your Baby Become a Better Sleeper

It's not unusual for a newborn to wake Mom and Dad half a dozen times a night. In fact, it typically takes them three to six months to stretch those nighttime naps into four to six-hour durations. Until they get to that point, there are some things you can do to encourage better, longer cycles.

Much like adults, babies sleep better in total darkness. This helps their body to know that it is nighttime, which also means sleep time. By getting some block-out curtains and dimming the lights, your baby's body will set itself into "sleep mode."

Having a routine will also help your baby's body get used to getting sleepy around the same time every day. Like your body would indicate to you that it is getting tired around the time that you go to bed every night, your baby's body will work in the same way. This is the same scenario with daytime naps.

Many parents testify that giving a warm bath, singing lullabies, and reading books help get your baby nice and sleepy before bed. These are all ways to calm them and give them a reset from the busy day. It can also alert them to know that sleep is to follow.

Before your baby can roll, you can also swaddle them. To swaddle your baby, you need to lay a blanket on the bed (or a flat, even surface) with one of the corners facing upward, making the blanket into a diamond shape. You then need to fold the top corner over and place your baby down on their back, with their head positioned just above the folded line. From there, you will fold the right side of the blanket over your baby and tuck the end under the left side of your baby's back. You can then fold up the bottom corner of the diamond over your baby. The last step is to fold the left corner over your baby, toward the right-hand side. Make sure you wrap them up nice and snug so that they feel secure. Once your baby can roll over, it is best to avoid swaddling as their hands will not be able to help them lift up if they roll onto their tummies.

While these tips will prove to help your baby get better sleep in the long term, it is important to remain patient. These techniques will not magically work overnight, so give it time and remember the end goal.

Steps to Creating a Sleep-Friendly Routine and Environment

Even as adults, our routine leading up to bedtime can have a significant impact on the quality of our sleep. If you have been to a party and immediately try to fall asleep when you get home, chances are that you will struggle to settle your mind; and even if your body gets to rest, you will wake up feeling mentally tired. The same applies to babies. You have to remember that they too have emotions, thoughts, and fluctuating energy levels. By ticking off some good habits throughout the day, you will be setting your baby (and yourself) up for a better night's sleep.

- **Be intentional with the routine that you would like to have with your baby.** Start by introducing sleep habits that will give your baby their cue that it's almost bedtime.

- **Plan out a bedtime routine.** Ask yourself, what would be realistically possible for you to do with your baby every night before they go to bed and implement it.

- **Try to stick to a bedtime.** Babies thrive on routines so choose a time that will be convenient for them to go down for the night and try to stick to it.

- **Create a safe and practical sleep environment.** You want your baby to feel at ease and secure in the place where they will spend the night.

- **Make sure that your baby is not overtired or overstimulated.** By encouraging them to take frequent naps during the day, you will get them at the right window for sleeping through.

- **Feed your baby frequently during the day.** The most common reason for babies waking up is hunger, so make sure that they are nice and full come nighttime to minimize the amount of times that they wake up.

Once again, these steps will be a work in progress. You might have some trial and error, but if you go through each step you will be working toward good nighttime habits that have a positive long-term impact.

Managing Sleep Regressions and Transitions

"Sleep Regression" is a term that many parents dread hearing. You are barely getting any sleep, so how is it possible that it could be regressing? Why is it regressing? You just got into a good sleeping habit. Well, first of all, sleep regressions are completely normal and very common in babies. The most obvious sign that your baby is going through a sleep regression is if they were sleeping fairly well and all of a sudden, they start waking up every couple of hours.

Regressions are the most common at around the four-month mark and then again when your baby starts reaching big milestones. For example, when your baby learns how to sit up from a lying down position, you might find that they will be all too eager to practice this new skill in the middle of the night.

Do not panic too soon though as regressions will usually only last a week or two and your child will be back on track. It is crucial, however, that you stick to good habits during this time. If you fall into bad sleep habits during a regression, such as nursing your baby to sleep every time they wake up, you will very quickly get your baby used to this new routine.

Tips on How to Cope With Sleep Regressions

To help you continue on a good path toward sleeping through the night while you are in the regression phase, here are a few key tips:

- **Use this time to ace your sleep training method.** Your baby will be waking up more frequently, will be harder to put to sleep, and will be a bit fussier, so take this more difficult time to instill the long-term method that you want your baby to fall asleep to.

- **Stick to your routine.** As tempting as it may be, now is not the time to abandon the routine that you have worked so hard to achieve. Continue with it to your best ability and your baby will eventually fall in line again.

- **Make sure you feed your baby frequently throughout the day so that they have less chance of waking up during the night due to hunger.** At this stage, their sleep will be very light so any small feeling of discomfort will disturb them.

- **Ensure that your baby is getting enough stimulation during the day.** If your baby is bored and not being stimulated, this can lead to a bad night's sleep.

- **By the four-month mark, you should be able to know what your baby's sleep cues are.** By identifying these and starting the sleep routine on time, you will minimize the risk of your baby becoming overtired and refusing sleep.

- **Remember to take care of yourself.** You will need a lot of patience and calmness when going through a regression so that you can deal with it correctly. If you do not take care of yourself, you will have a very hard time going through this.

The best part about a regression is that it is not a long-term issue and, when handled correctly, it will go away just as quickly as it appeared.

Transitioning From Co-Sleeping to Independent Sleep

If you start with a co-sleeping arrangement with your baby, then you will eventually want them to move to a more independent sleeping setup.

You may want to stop co-sleeping once your baby starts rolling around in their sleep, or if it starts to hinder your sleep instead of helping you sleep better through the night. If your baby is a light sleeper, you may end up waking them up every time that you move.

Some babies may be very easygoing and can immediately settle into a new routine once they are moved into their own room. But, for the most part, babies will need time to adapt. There are a few things that you can do to make this transition more bearable and sustainable.

Bring Your Child's Crib Into Your Room

If your baby will be transitioning from a Moses Basket or newborn sleeper to a bigger crib, then start by getting them used to sleeping in their crib next to you or in the location of their previous "bed." Once they are used to their new crib in your room, you can work on moving it further away.

Gradually Increase the Space

If your baby has separation anxiety, it will be best to work on getting them further and further away from you gradually. Start by moving their crib a bit further away from your bed and increase this space by a little bit every day, eventually leading to their own room.

Move Into Your Child's Room

If possible, try moving into your child's room temporarily. You are your child's safe space and comfort. It can give them quite a shock if they are used to sleeping close to you, in your room, and suddenly they are in another room far away from you. Try spending as much time in their new room with them as possible and sit close by while they fall asleep.

Familiarize Your Child With Their New Space

New parents tend to do everything in the main bedroom for the first few months and when the baby finally transitions to the nursery, it is an unfamiliar room to them which makes the move all the more difficult.

Even if the newborn is sleeping in your bedroom, try to spend some time during the day in the nursery so that your baby can start looking around and recognizing the space. You can change diapers, play, read, and sing. Make sure that you create a positive and pleasant atmosphere so that when your baby finally transitions, they have good memories and feelings about the space.

Try It for Nap Times

Start your child off by having their day naps in their new room and crib so that they can get used to spending longer stretches there when they transition to nighttime sleep. You can use naptime to begin sleep training in their new space and by the time you move them to their new room permanently, they will be used to the routine and methods that you have set up for their sleep.

Through all of these tips, the main goal is that your babies learn that they must fall asleep in their beds, in their rooms. To get them used to this idea, you will have to repeat these steps frequently no matter how tired you are at night or how many times your baby has awakened. Babies can learn new habits very quickly, so if you persist and remain consistent, your baby will soon realize that this is their new norm.

There is no ideal or recommended age to start the transition to the baby's room, so this will be entirely dependent on your family's needs.

Managing Nap Schedules and Sleep Associations

While each baby can be vastly different, some general guidelines for naps can help your baby develop healthy sleep habits. Naps—and sleep in general—are vital to a baby's growth and development. Not to mention that it will give you some time to catch up on sleep and work around the house.

The issue is that babies can be very fussy sleepers. In the early days, they do not consume large amounts of food which leads them to be hungry very often, day and night. Add gas, colic, and light sleep to the mix and you have a baby who is very hard to put to sleep and stay asleep.

A key to having a good sleeper by 12 months of age is to develop good sleeping habits from the start and have your child follow a sleep routine that is suitable to their age. A guideline to how often your baby should be sleeping is as follows:

- **Newborn (0 to 6 weeks):** Newborns are asleep most of the time and only stay awake for a window of about an hour and a half. This time is usually spent feeding, burping, and changing them. They will then usually sleep for a period of two to four hours at a time, both day and night.

- **Two to three months old:** At this age, your baby might start forming a pattern with their sleep. If not, that is also completely normal! Most babies will have about three daytime naps, ranging from half an hour to three hours long. Babies who have short naps might still require a fourth nap during the day. You can also move the baby's bedtime to earlier in the evening (the general recommendation is around seven).

- **Four to six months old:** By now, your baby should be well on their way to having a routine and sleep association. The good news: Sleeping through the night may not be that far away. Your baby should be taking about three naps by this point and sleeping for approximately 10 hours at night. This might not yet be 10 hours straight, but you are approaching that stage. It is important to remember that naps are still very much essential to ensure a happy baby and a good night's sleep. Many parents fall into the trap of thinking that if they keep their baby awake for most of the day, they will sleep through the night; however, with babies, the opposite is true. Babies who are overtired and overstimulated will wake up frequently throughout the night and will be restless, cranky, and difficult to deal with. Many moms will be going back to work during these months. If that is the case, it's important to advise your child's caregiver on the methods that you have set up for their nap times.

Another thing to keep in mind in this age group is the possible sleep regression. Remember that you must just remain calm and consistent if your child goes through the four-month sleep regression.

- **Six to ten months:** Between six and ten months of age, many babies start sleeping through the night. That is cause for celebration! However, there is still a lot going on with your baby's development, so it cannot be guaranteed that every night will be a good one. While it will be exciting in your baby's life for the amount of new skills that they will be learning, it is also a big reason why your baby will be overstimulated, which leads to them having a bit more difficulty settling down and sleeping at night.

You might find your baby practicing rolling or sitting up in the middle of the night. Apart from all the new skills, babies older than six months will also start realizing that they are separate from their mother or primary caregiver, which can lead to separation anxiety. You may find that every time you try to put them down, they will wake up and cry. They will want you very close a lot of the time.

Your baby might transition to a morning nap and an afternoon nap only; however, some babies might still have three naps split up into a morning nap, an afternoon nap, and a catnap in the early evening. The longer naps should not exceed two hours and the catnap nap should be about 30 minutes.

- **Ten to twelve months:** These last few months will be the most crucial in setting your baby up for good nighttime sleep through their toddler years. Your baby should have learned very good habits at this stage. By now, they will most likely be having two long (about two-hour) naps during the day. If you did sleep training, then your baby should be able to be put down while awake and settle themselves to sleep, and they should be sleeping through the night. Sounds like a dream come true, doesn't it? Well, it is. But, babies are still human beings and not robots so there are a few bumps that you might encounter.

  At this age, babies are very social and do not want to miss out. This might make it quite hard, if almost impossible, to settle a baby if you are out and about. They are also learning a lot of new things including walking and saying a few words. Why would they want to sleep when they have a lot of learning and development to do? This is where all of the training that you have done up to this point will come into play. If you have and continue to remain consistent with sleep associations and routines, bedtimes and nap times should be easier to manage.

- **Twelve months:** By this time, some babies might start to fool you into thinking that they are ready to transition to one nap only. But, they are still too young for this and you will find yourself struggling with nighttime sleep or having a cranky toddler if you allow this to happen. Instead, wake them up earlier in the morning so that they are tired enough to squeeze in a quick nap in the late morning and then another in the afternoon.

Parent Self-Care and Sleep Hygiene

Sleep deprivation is no joke, and it can make even the most resilient parent crumble. This is not something that you can prepare for and is not something that you have done before. Sure, maybe you spent a week camping and barely slept, but the difference is that you were able to catch up on that lost sleep. When you have a baby, you are sleep-deprived for months at a time and there are very limited chances to catch up on that. This is a big adjustment and can lead to a dip in your productivity, as well as your mood.

Although your main goal right now is to care for your baby, it's vital that you remember that your baby (and the entire household for that matter) cannot function if you are unwell or stressed out. You need to take care of yourself in order to be able to take care of others. This may be easier said than done, but there are a couple of things you can try to help.

Firstly, it's important that you ask for help. Whether this is to look after the baby while you catch up on some rest or help with some chores around the house, friends and family will be all too happy to lend a helping hand if this means that they get to spend a bit of time with the baby in exchange.

Right now, you might be trying to live off of caffeine, but it's essential that you make healthy choices when it comes to your diet. You may crave sugary foods due to your energy levels being low, but this will not sustain you in the long run. You may also want to spend time scrolling on your phone or watching videos online when your baby is sleeping, but this will only leave you more exhausted. As much as you are craving the "me-time" and a bit of normalcy, try to put rest first and your phone later.

Coping With Postpartum Sleep Changes

Apart from the fact that your baby is waking up frequently during the night, your body will also go through some postpartum changes that can affect your sleep. These include changes to your iron levels and hormones, as well as a general readjustment of your body. You might also be in some pain from the birthing process and could be on painkillers or other medication. This all plays a role in your body lacking the sleep that you ought to be getting. Try to rest as much as possible and talk to your doctor about taking an iron supplement to help increase your energy levels as naturally as possible.

It does not come as a surprise to know that you will be sleep-deprived when you have a baby. This is probably one of the most well-known aspects: babies are not great sleepers, especially at night. While this is completely normal and to be expected, there are some ways in which you can train your child or resources that you can invest in to make life easier during these first few months. Remember that it will get easier the older the baby gets!

Another factor to ensure that your child sleeps well is their hunger levels. Full babies tend to sleep better. In the next chapter, we can explore how you can ensure that your child is well-fed, which leads to contentment and better sleep!

Help Transform Lives with Your Review

Embrace the Power of Generosity

"Money can't buy happiness but giving it away can." - Freddie Mercury

Would you extend a helping hand to someone you've never met, even without seeking recognition for it?

Who is this person, you ask? They are akin to who you once were—less experienced, eager to make a difference, and seeking guidance without knowing where to find it.

Our mission is to make the journey of new parents accessible to everyone. Everything we do stems from that mission. And the only way for us to accomplish that mission is by reaching... well... everyone.

This is where you come in. Most people judge a book by its cover (and its reviews). **So please consider helping that new parent by leaving a review for "*The Newborn Parenting Guide (Made Easy)*" by Nicole Stanton.** Your gift costs no money and takes less than 60 seconds to make a real impact, yet it can change a fellow parent's life forever. Your review could help... Leave a review to experience the satisfaction of genuinely helping someone in need.

Scan the QR code below to leave your review:

Thank you from the bottom of my heart. Now, let's get back to helping one another navigate the joys and challenges of parenthood.

Your biggest supporter, Nicole Stanton

Chapter 7:

Feeding and Nutrition

Anything can start to taste good if you have enough positive memories of being fed it by a parent. —Bee Wilson

When it comes to feeding your newborn, experts agree that nature provides the best nourishment. Breast milk contains all the nutrition your baby needs. In fact, it changes consistency and modifies nutritional needs as your baby grows. It's easy on their digestive system too. Healthy fats, proteins, and sugars are readily absorbed, and few issues occur unless Mom passes along something that disagrees with them. For example, gas-producing food like broccoli may cause your baby uncomfortable tummy bubbles.

Breastfeeding is not always an option, though. Some women may have had their ducts removed during a mastectomy for cancer treatment. Others may find it difficult, painful, or otherwise unhealthy for them to continue. Sometimes, the amount of milk produced is insufficient. Many women prefer the convenience of formula. Though not as nutritionally complete, infant formulas provide an excellent alternative to breast milk.

In this chapter, we'll discuss the pros and cons of breastfeeding and formula feeding. We'll also talk about introducing solid foods to your baby, navigating feeding challenges, and promoting long-term healthy eating habits.

Breastfeeding and Formula-Feeding

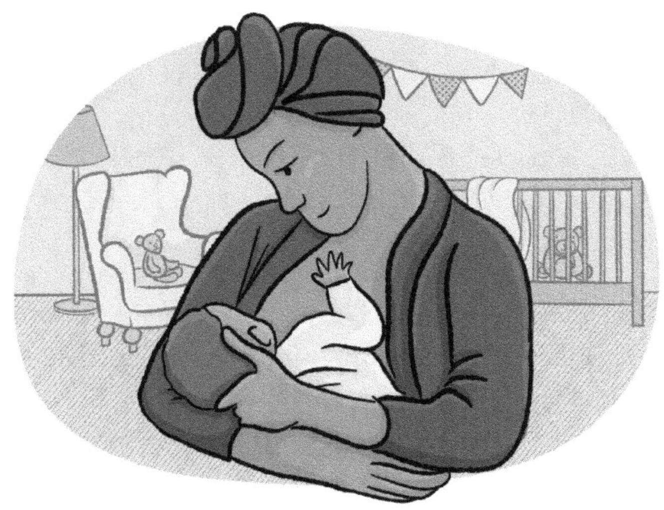

Breast milk and formula are both viable feeding options for your newborn. Both have their own perks as well as a few drawbacks. Let's take a look at breastfeeding first.

Breastfeeding

Before your baby is born—as early as your fourth week of pregnancy—your body begins the process of making their food. Milk-producing tissues called lactocytes grow at this stage, causing tenderness and enlargement of the breasts. Actual milk will not be expressed or released, however, until the baby is born.

Once you deliver your child, pregnancy hormones will drop, and prolactin—the lactation hormone—will increase. Prolactin and your baby's suckling will stimulate your breasts to produce milk. Oxytocin is also released when the baby nurses, causing breast muscles to contract and push the milk through the ducts. This is referred to as "let-down," and it is a sensation you will feel when it is time to nurse.

Breast milk goes through three different stages, as described below:

- **Colostrum:** Your first milk is a thick, sticky, yellowish substance that is high in white blood cells and antibodies. It contains the same nutrients as later-stage milk and is tailored by nature to suit your newborn.

- **Transitional:** Two to four days after giving birth, your breast milk will become creamier, with high levels of fat, lactose, protein, and vitamins. This is referred to as your milk "coming in." Your breasts may feel fuller and firmer during this stage.

- **Mature:** About 10–15 days after delivery, your milk will change its consistency once more, becoming thinner and whiter, but still full of nutrients. The composition, however, may change from day to day, depending on the child's needs. For example, your body may generate antibiotics to pass along to the baby to help them fight illness. Breast milk consistency may also change during a feeding.

  - **Fore milk:** This milk comes out of the breast first. It is thin and watery to quench the baby's thirst.

  - **Hind milk:** This follows the fore milk and is thicker, higher in fat, contains more calories, and satisfies the baby's hunger.

Breast milk will remain in the mature stage until you wean for the baby. Keep in mind that infants' feeding needs will change as they grow. *Healthline* provides the below chart to help you know what to expect (Christiano, 2023):

- **From birth to 3 months:** Your newborn will nurse 7 to 9 times every 24 hours.

- **From 3 months to 6 months:** Your baby will nurse 6 to 8 times every 24 hours.

- **From 6 months to 12 months:** Your baby will nurse about 6 times every 24 hours; solid foods are introduced.

- **At 12 months:** The frequency of nursing may reduce to around 4 times a day, as your baby incorporates more solid foods into their diet, which keep them fuller and fulfill nutritional needs.

Pros and Cons of Breastfeeding:

Johns Hopkins Medicine (n.d.-a) recommends breastfeeding for a minimum of six months and continuing for up to two years. The longer you nurse, the greater the health benefits you and your child will receive.

Here are some breastfeeding perks for Mom:

- It speeds up pregnancy weight loss.

- It lowers your risk of diabetes and obesity.

- It contracts and shrinks your uterus to pre-pregnant size.

- It reduces the risk of breast and ovarian cancer.

- It saves you $2,000–$4,000 annually, compared to the cost of formula (Porter, 2018).

Your baby will benefit from breast milk in the following ways:

- It strengthens your baby's immunity, reduces the frequency of infections, and lessens the severity of illnesses.

- It helps prevent allergies, asthma, and certain childhood cancers.

- It lowers the risk of SIDS, obesity, and diabetes.

- It contributes to higher-quality long-term health.

- It improves eye function, stimulates brain growth, and develops the nervous system.

- It increases water content to provide extra hydration when the baby is sick.

- It automatically adjusts to the right temperature and is never too hot or too cold.

While, nutrition-wise, nothing beats breast milk, the act of breastfeeding has some disadvantages:

- **Engorgement:** Your breasts will fill with milk when it's time to feed the baby. Sometimes, this can be very uncomfortable, and you may experience breast tightness or firmness. Frequent nursing will help relieve the discomfort.

- **Leakage:** If you are not able to nurse when your breasts are full, they may leak until you feed the baby or pump the milk. Leakage occurs less frequently over time as your body adjusts to the baby's feeding schedule. In the meantime, you may want to purchase cloth or disposable nursing pads to protect your clothing.

- **Breast pain and sore nipples:** It can take a few days for you and your baby to get the hang of breastfeeding. Though your body was designed by nature to do this task, if it's never done the job before, it might require a little practice. Much like how your muscles ache when you begin a new fitness routine, your breasts and nipples may be sore and sensitive for a while.

- **Inconvenience:** If you return to work or leave the house for an extended time, you will need to pump before you leave and possibly while you're away. Some women find this inconvenient, but others don't seem to mind, as long as they can keep the supply refrigerated or frozen for later use.

- **Exhaustion:** According to the Western Missouri Medical Center, 25% of the body's energy is consumed by breast milk. They go on to say that the metabolic energy required for you to breastfeed a baby every day is the same amount you use by walking seven miles (Porter, 2018). That's quite a workout! No wonder you're more tired, thirstier, and hungrier than usual.

For a variety of reasons, some newborns are unable to breastfeed immediately. Below are some alternative feeding methods used for a temporary transition:

- **Cup:** Cup feeding is used for infants who reject a bottle nipple or who have trouble latching. To cup feed, hold your baby upright and offer a small, half-full cup of breast milk to their lips. Do not pour the liquid into their mouth, but allow them to lap it with their tongue.

- **Spoon:** Similar to cup feeding, but in a more manageable container. Offer one spoonful of breast milk at a time to your baby's lips and allow them to lap it with their tongue.

- **Syringe:** This option is less likely to spill. Fill a medicine syringe with breast milk and gently ease a very small bit into your baby's mouth at a time.

- **Finger:** This technique is used for infants who have a difficult time suckling. A tube extends from a bottle or cup of breast milk and is adhered to your finger. Gently insert your finger with the tube into their mouth, and as they suck, milk will flow through the tube into their mouth.

- **Lactation aid:** Similar to finger-feeding, a tube extends from a bottle or cup but is adhered to your breast. As the baby suckles, they get a supplemental flow, and the action encourages more production from you.

- **Paced bottle feeding:** This method is often used for babies born preterm and by mothers who are returning to work or school. The infant is offered a bottle with a slow-flowing nipple and is allowed to suck 5-10 times and is then given a break. If they are still interested in feeding, return the bottle to their lips and repeat the process. This method helps prevent overfeeding because it teaches the baby to listen to their natural hunger cues and stop when satisfied rather than parents encouraging them to drink until the bottle is empty.

Best Ways to Hold Your Baby While You Breastfeed

There are several different positions in which to hold your baby while you nurse. You may find that certain positions encourage the baby to suckle more or that other positions are too comfortable and make them fall asleep before they are full. It's a good idea to try a few holds to see what's most comfortable for both of you.

Below are some common ways to hold your baby while you breastfeed:

- **Cradle position:** Hold the baby with their head on your forearm and their body snugly facing yours.

- **Cross-cradle:** Hold the baby across your chest and support their head with the palm of your hand at the base of their neck. This position is helpful for premature babies or those who have a weak suckling action.

- **Football hold:** Hold the baby in a more upright position along your side with their head at nipple-level and keep the palm of your hand at the base of their neck.

- **Straddle:** Lie back on a pillow and place the baby's head between your breasts. Allow the baby to search out the breast and latch on naturally.

- **Side-lying:** Lie on your side with the baby facing you and pull them close, facing your body, and encourage them to latch. This position is comfortable for women who've had C-sections as it keeps the baby's pressure and weight off their abdomen while they heal.

You may also choose to purchase a nursing pillow, which provides support for the baby and comfort for both of you while you nurse.

Common Breastfeeding Concerns and Challenges

Many first-time moms aren't sure what to expect when it comes to breastfeeding. Though it's a natural process, it's not something you do all the time!

Some common breastfeeding challenges are below:

- **Painful or intense let-down:** When your breasts are too full, they can feel tight and sore. If you experience a tingling or pin-prick sensation, this could indicate infection, and you should contact your healthcare provider.

- **Too much milk:** The more frequently you nurse, the more milk your breasts will produce. Try going longer breaks between feedings to slow production.

- **Too little milk:** As noted above, milk production is supply and demand. Too little milk can indicate you are not feeding often enough. Try to nurse more frequently or pump between feedings to stimulate more production.

- **Plugged milk ducts:** This can occur when one or more ducts don't drain properly. To encourage it to loosen and release, breastfeed only on that side and make sure your bra is not too tight.

- **Large, flat, or inverted nipples:** Some women's body structure may make it challenging to breastfeed. However, it's not impossible! It may take the baby a couple of weeks to learn to latch onto large nipples, but they will get the hang of it as long as your milk production is sufficient. For flat or inverted nipples, the baby must latch onto both the nipple and the breast. Often, over time, the nipple will protrude with the baby's consistent sucking.

- **Breast infection (mastitis):** Mastitis is an infection in your breast that usually occurs only one at a time. It can give you flu-like symptoms, including a fever, nausea, and vomiting, and it may cause a yellowish discharge from the infected breast. It often clears by itself within 48 hours, but if it doesn't, consult your physician for treatment.

- **Thrush:** Thrush is a fungal infection caused by an overgrowth of candida, or yeast. It is usually spread from the baby's mouth to your breast and can result in painful cracked, peeling, and blistered nipples. Consult your physician for treatment and your child's pediatrician to clear their infection as well. Change nursing pads frequently, wear a clean bra every day, and wash your hands and your baby's hands frequently.

- **Baby refuses to nurse:** Sometimes, babies will suddenly seem to lose interest in breastfeeding. They may turn away or cry and resist all your efforts. This usually indicates painful teething or a possible illness, like an ear infection or something else that is causing them discomfort. Pump your milk to prevent engorgement and assess the baby's health. Try different nursing positions, feed the baby in a quiet environment, and consult your pediatrician if necessary.

Weaning

Doctors recommend solely breastfeeding or formula-feeding your baby for the first six months. Breast milk and formula provide all the nutrition they need during that time, and their digestive system is not ready to process other substances. At six months, if you are ready to stop breastfeeding, you can switch to formula but do not give your child cow's milk until they are 12 months old or older.

There is no set time to stop nursing your baby. When you stop depends on you and your child. If you're both comfortable and everything's going well, you can continue until your child is two or older.

Below are some options for a successful, low-stress weaning process:

- Eliminate one feeding per day, and gradually taper off completely. Nurse after your child has a snack or meal if they're older so they drink less during that session. Shorten the time of the feeding each day until that one has been dropped. Gradual weaning helps your supply slowly reduce and can prevent engorgement and plugged ducts.

- Partially wean. Offer to nurse at certain times of the day and give your child a bottle during the others. For example, breastfeed overnight but not during the day, or breastfeed in the morning but not in the afternoon. You can use pumped breast milk in the bottles, formula, or cow's milk if your baby is older than 12 months.

- If you're weaning a younger baby, use bottle nipples that are designed for preemies and have a slow flow.

- If your baby resists the change, have your spouse or caregiver feed them instead of you.

Formula Feeding

While breastfeeding is the best choice nutritionally, it isn't the right option for everyone. If you've had a mastectomy due to cancer, or if you have damaged or injured breast tissue, you may be physically unable to nurse. In addition, your physician may advise you to stop breastfeeding if you're not producing a sufficient amount of milk, an infection has passed from you to your baby, or you are taking certain medications that have been transferred through your milk and are harming the baby. Recreational drugs and alcohol can also be transmitted to the baby via breast milk, so mothers of newborns who engage in such activity should not breastfeed either. Some women simply prefer bottle feeding because they find breastfeeding uncomfortable and difficult, or because it is more convenient for their spouse and caregivers.

Whether you bottle feed by choice or necessity, you should speak to your pediatrician beforehand. Based on your child's weight, size, and overall health, your doctor can advise which formula will have the best benefits for your baby's specific needs. They can also advise how many ounces you should offer at various stages of growth.

Below, we'll talk about when to introduce the bottle to your infant, the different formulas available, and the pros and cons of bottle feeding.

Introducing the Bottle

Doctors recommend introducing your baby to the bottle whether or not you use formula because you will use bottles to feed the baby pumped breast milk. If you are breastfeeding first, you should wait at least six weeks to give the baby a bottle, or they may refuse the breast. Of course, you'll need a bottle right from the start if you won't be breastfeeding at all. Consult the hospital nursery staff about the formula they have on hand and ask for samples they can send home with you.

Choosing Your Baby Formula

Infant formula can be purchased in powder form that you measure and mix with water, liquid concentrate that also needs to be measured and mixed with water, and ready-to-feed liquid.

According to Dr. Bridget Young of *Healthline* (2022), fat, protein, and carbohydrates make up about 98% of all formulas. Other label ingredients are not regulated or essential to your infant's health. Below is an explanation of the proteins and carbohydrates in the formula to help you choose what's right for your little one:

- **Protein:** Infant formulas are either cow milk-based or soy-based. The size of the proteins is what's important. Standard formulas contain large, full-sized proteins that most infants can process. However, babies with digestion issues or who have difficulty breaking down large proteins may need a formula with either partially or fully hydrolyzed protein. That means that the proteins have been broken apart and made smaller so they are easier to digest. Fully hydrolyzed proteins are extremely small and are considered hypoallergenic. These formulas should be given to babies with cow milk allergies or severe digestive issues.

- **Carbohydrates:** Both breast and dairy milk contain lactose, which most infants can digest. The digestive tracts of some infants, however, produce an insufficient amount of the enzyme that breaks down lactose, so it may be a good idea to switch to a soy-based formula or a lactose-reduced option that contains sucrose or glucose if that is the case.

Of special note, Dr. Young recommends using whey protein formulas for babies with acid reflux. She also says that palm oil in formula is known to cause constipation, and partially hydrolyzed whey protein in formula improves baby eczema.

Healthline provides this list of the 7 best formulas on the market, organized by how each one benefits your baby (Marcin & Dix, 2023):

- **Best overall:** Bobbie Organic Infant Formula

- **Most similar to breast milk:** Enfamil Gentlease Infant Formula

- **Most budget-friendly:** Kirkland Signature ProCare Baby Formula

- **Best for preemies:** Similac NeoSure Infant Formula

- **Best plant-based formula:** Gerber Good Start Soy Powder Infant Formula

- **Best for food allergies:** Enfamil Nutramigen with Enflora LGG Infant Formula

- **Best name-brand formula:** Similac 360 Total Care Infant Formula

The American Association of Pediatrics provides the following schedule to help you know how often your baby will feed and how much your baby will drink per feeding during their first year (Jain, 2023):

- They will drink only .5 ounces in the first few days, and will then increase to 1–3 ounces.

- At about 2 months, they will drink 4–5 ounces every 3–4 hours.

- At 4 months, they will take about 4–6 ounces about every 4 hours.

- At 6 months, they will drink up to 8 ounces every 4–6 hours.

- From 6 to 12 months, they will continue to drink about 8 ounces, but the frequency may decrease as you introduce solid foods into their diet.

Positions for Bottle Feeding

You'll want to hold your baby in a position that is comfortable for both of you and enhances the baby's feeding experience. Below are some common options:

- **Cradle:** Rest your baby's head in the crook of your arm and tilt it slightly at an angle. This position is great for skin-to-skin time.

- **Feeding pillow:** Give your arms a little break and allow the pillow to support the baby. You will still need to hold the bottle with your other hand.

- **Sitting position:** Sit down and hold the baby in a seated position with their back against your chest. Be sure to keep the bottle tipped at an appropriate angle.

- **Baby on your legs:** Sit or lie down with your legs bent at the knee. Place the baby on their back on your thighs and offer them a bottle. This is great to encourage interaction and eye contact.

Pros and Cons of Formula Feeding

The top perk of formula feeding is that Mom's not the only one who can feed the baby! Dad, grandparents, and other caregivers can give the baby a bottle and take a little work off your responsibilities. Below are some other benefits:

- It is fast and easy to prepare.

- You don't have to guess how much the baby drank because it's been measured out.

- You can offer more if the baby's still hungry without wondering about your breast milk supply.

- Bottle feeding causes no physical discomfort to you.

- Formula-fed babies often stay fuller longer than breast milk-fed infants.

- Formula-fed babies sleep through the night sooner than breastmilk-fed infants.

- Other people can help out and bond with the baby.

Of course, there are some drawbacks of bottle feeding too:

- Your baby does not as easily digest or as effectively process formula as they do breast milk.

- There is a higher risk for formula-fed babies to develop milk allergies.

- Your baby's gut bacteria can be altered by formula and lead to diarrhea and discomfort.

- Formula, bottles, and other equipment can be very expensive.

- Bottles can leak, and nipples can tear.

- Bacteria can grow and make your child ill if bottles and nipples are not completely clean and sterile.

Whichever feeding method you choose, make sure you are supplying your baby the nutrition they need.

Introducing Solid Foods

As your child grows older and is introduced to solid food and liquids other than milk, their nutrient requirements and the amount of milk produced will change. Keep in mind that though you may incorporate solid foods into their diet, your baby will still get the majority of the nutrition they need from breastmilk or formula until 12 months of age. You are adding to their diet, not making any replacements.

The Centers for Disease Control and Prevention (CDC) recommends introducing solid foods to your infant when they are no younger than six months of age. The following signs will help you know when your child is ready for the transition (2023):

- They can sit up by themselves or with support.

- They can hold up and control the motion and stability of their head and neck.

- They put objects in or move things toward their mouth.

- They can grasp and hold toys, food, and other small objects.

- They open their mouth if you offer food.

- They move food to the back of the mouth with their tongue to swallow.

- They swallow food instead of spitting it back out.

If you introduce solid foods at six months, by your child's seventh or eighth, they can eat a wide variety of foods, like infant cereals and pureed fruits vegetables, meats, cheese, and yogurt. The CDC (2020d) recommends varying the infant cereals (barley, oats, and multi-grain) to avoid overexposure to arsenic by feeding them only the rice meal. All of these items can be purchased at your local grocer, but if you choose to prepare them at home yourself, remove all seeds, stems, pits, skin, fat, and bones and then cook the ingredients until they can be mashed with a fork. You can add breast milk or formula to make a creamy consistency that may be more palatable until your baby is ready for thicker textures.

Give your baby only one single nutrient food at a time over 3–5 days to make sure your child has no adverse reactions to it before trying a new food. Common food allergens to watch out for include peanuts and tree nuts, cow's milk, eggs, soy, sesame, fish, shellfish, and wheat. Honey can contain botulism spores, so do not offer it until after your child's first birthday. Also, do not give your child finger foods until they are at least 8-10 months old. It helps if they have some teeth. At this point, you can finely chop soft fruits, vegetables, and fully cooked meats, as well as pasta, crackers, and dry cereal.

In Summary

Many comedians have joked that all babies do is eat, sleep, and need clean diapers. We laugh at that sentiment because there's a lot of truth to it, at least for their first few months of life. In this chapter, we talked a lot about your baby's nutritional needs and how to satisfy them safely and sufficiently. We looked at your options for breastfeeding and formula feeding and considered the pros and cons of each. We also learned about weaning and introducing solid foods.

In the following chapter, we'll delve into childproofing your home to ensure optimal safety and well-being.

Chapter 8:

Safety and Childproofing

There is no greater warrior than a mother protecting her child. —N.K. Jemisin

The best way to test whether your house is childproof is to get an actual child in there, you will be able to pick up in less than an hour what will need to change when your little one arrives. I once had a childless friend tell me that her house was totally childproofed. Let's just say that a lot happened including a freestanding mirror falling over! Adults' minds have been programmed to know what we should and shouldn't do, touch, or play with. However a child is a clean slate, and babies and toddlers are even more so. They have no concept of electricity or how dangerous it can be. All they know is that there are tiny holes all over the walls that are the perfect size for their little fingers to go in and at just the right height too!

It is unrealistic to expect an exploring baby or even a toddler to know better and to stay clear of dangerous things. That is why it is our duty as parents and caregivers to set up the house in a way that will keep them safe and protected, and above all, will remove dangerous temptation from them.

In 2021, an estimated 175,500 preventable injury-related deaths occurred in homes and communities, or about 78% of all preventable injury-related deaths that year. The number of deaths was up 12.3% from the 2020 total of 156,300. An additional 52,500,000 people suffered nonfatal medically consulted injuries. The death rate per 100,000 population was 52.9—about 12.2% higher than the 2020 rate. (NSC, n.d.).

Home Safety Essentials

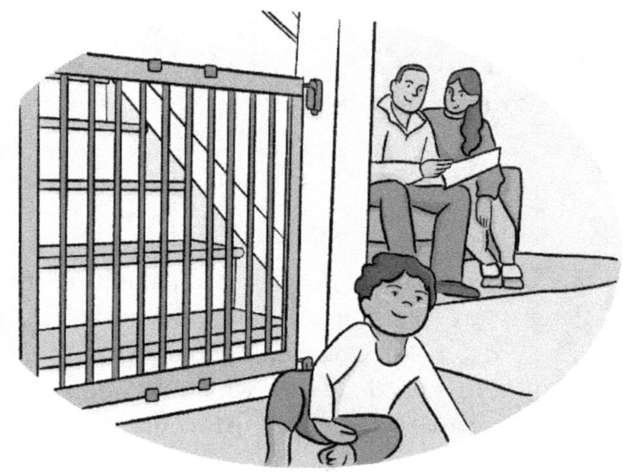

When baby-proofing your home or surroundings, try to think of the most common ways that babies can be injured. Think along the lines of choking, falling, electrocution, strangling, and poisoning.

While an adult should always be around to supervise, it is best to ensure that your home is as baby-proof as possible to ensure any accidents if you are temporarily distracted, gone to the bathroom, or when the baby becomes more mobile and explores.

Falling

It can take babies a while to be stable when they are sitting or standing. Even when they start sitting independently at around 6 months of age, you will quickly notice that they won't be able to be put on a chair with no securing mechanism and stay put. They will most likely bend forward and fall off. Whenever you place them in a chair, car seat, or any similar designs, make sure that they are securely fastened in.

Stairs should have a toddler-proof security gate and babies and toddlers should only go up and down the stairs when you or any other adult supervisor is with them.

Parents usually find out that their baby can roll once they have rolled themselves off the bed and landed on the floor. Sometimes you may not know that your baby has learned or reached a particular milestone until they just do it out of the blue. You should always be prepared and ensure that they are blocked from falling off the bed by using cushions instead of assuming and having your baby injured.

Poisoning

Poisoning is one of the most common accidental injuries that can happen to children. Parents are often totally unaware until it is too late. The reason for this is that most households keep their cleaning products under the sink in an unlocked cabinet which can be easily accessible to crawling or walking babies. Move all of your cleaning detergents to cabinets that are higher up or install a lock on the cabinet.

The same principle applies to medicine cabinets or other toiletries. Remember that a baby's natural reflex is to put whatever they pick up directly into their mouths. This goes for shampoos, lotions, oils, fabric softeners, and more.

If you have taken out a product to use, make sure that you put it back immediately as your little one will quickly spot it on the counter and realize that this is something new that they have not played with. If you are unable to pack and lock it away immediately, then at least make a mental note to place it high up.

Your child should know from a young age that medication and vitamins are only to be handled by adults. If you allow your baby to hold and play with bottles of medicine, even if very well sealed, they will not learn to treat this item as "out-of-bounds," and one day when you are not around, they may open it. Make sure that they know what items are to be left alone.

Lastly, always check the label for the recommended dosage of medication that your child must take. Do not give more than the prescribed or recommended amount.

Outdoor Safety

When choosing outdoor play equipment for your child, make sure that this is safe for your child and their age group. If your child is under the age of five, they should be supervised during outside playtime.

Many children get hurt while climbing, this can include jungle gyms and treehouses. Elevated trampolines that have no safety net could also prove to be a danger. Make sure that you watch your child and pick up on any areas for potential harm. Then try to child-proof those areas or teach your child how to navigate. If your child is a weak climber, it is unlikely that they will ever want to climb anything for the rest of their lives. So, teaching them how to do it correctly and safely would be the better option as opposed to avoiding it. Make sure that your child has supportive footwear with a good grip, or they could go barefoot and take the time to teach them.

One of the biggest, if not the biggest, outdoor hazards for small children is a swimming pool. Swimming pools can be extremely dangerous and it's important that you make sure it is child-proof as soon as you have your first child. Having a covering over the pool when it is not in use is a great way to ensure that your child cannot fall in, even if they are wandering about outside. If you decide to skip the covering and opt for a fence around the pool instead, it's vital that you check that it is closed properly before letting your child outside. There have been incidents of children letting their children into the garden and not knowing that a family member or garden service has left the pool gate open. By taking a few minutes to properly check this, you could be saving your child's life.

Basic First Aid Techniques

To get started with your first aid preparations, you will need to start with a first aid kit. The following items are recommended to keep on hand:

- pain and fever relief medication (paracetamol)

- thermometer

- bandages

- burn shields

- medicine pipette or dropper

- antiseptic ointment

- nasal aspirator

- constipation powder

- gripe water or gas drops

- allergy medication

With the help of your medical kit, there are a few first aid techniques that you should know and that will come in handy throughout your baby's childhood. Being able to react quickly could make the difference between the situation getting out of control or your child healing quickly.

Nose Bleeds

Help your child to sit back and keep their heads upright (try to avoid tilting the head back as this may lead to choking. Pinch the bridge of the nose gently for a couple of minutes for the bleeding to stop.

Try to also see what could have caused the bleeding to avoid it happening in the future. This can be from heat, stress, or it can just be genetics.

Wounds and Bruises

If your child has an open wound, the first step would be to apply pressure to the area to stop the bleeding. You can then wipe or dab the wound with a cotton ball dipped in lukewarm water and diluted antiseptic. Lastly, apply ointment and a bandage, depending on the size and severity of the wound.

Animal Bites and Stings

In the case of a sting, remove the stinger from the skin area immediately. Try to scrape the stinger out instead of pinching and pulling it out with your fingers as this may only release more venom. Then, wash the sting with soapy water and put pressure using a cold compress. You can then administer an allergy or paracetamol medication. Keep a close eye on your child for the next 24 hours to ensure that no severe allergic reaction takes place.

If your child has been bitten, the first step would be to apply pressure to the bite to stop any bleeding. You can then follow the same steps as you would to a wound. However, depending on the animal and the severity of the bite, you may need to take your child to get a tetanus vaccination.

Choking

This can be quite a scary one and quick thinking and action will definitely be required here! The first step would be to try to get your child to cough up the stuck item on their own. You should only give them a couple of seconds to try and then start the Heimlich maneuver. Do some research as to how to perform this safely depending on the age of your child as it may differ for smaller babies. Even if the item came out, it is still wise to go to your pediatrician for a check-up.

Head Injury

Start by checking the head for any visible bleeding or wound. Make sure that your child is able to clearly see you and comprehend what is going on. It is better to keep your child awake for at least an hour after the injury occurred. Keep checking on them for the next 24 hours and make sure that they can still walk with proper balance and do not have any signs of memory loss. If you are unsure, then head to the ER straight away.

Poisoning

You've caught your child with a bottle of bleach or detergent in their mouth, now what? You must act quickly and start by flushing the mouth out with water. Try to give them some milk to dilute the bleach and take them straight to the ER or pediatrician.

If your child has swallowed pills or medication then try to make them vomit it out before heading to the doctor.

In Summary

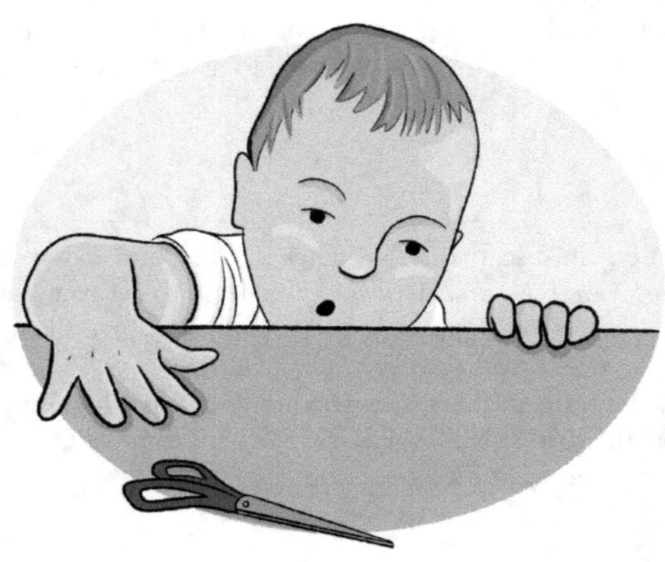

While this is, by far, not the part of parenting that people want to think about, it is a reality of life. Every parent wishes and hopes that no harm will come to their children, however, it is highly unlikely that they will make it to adulthood without a wound or bee sting at some point in their lives. Because most of these cannot be avoided, unless you place your child in a glass box, it's better that you read up and come to the incident prepared. Preparation can potentially save your child's life, or at least save on medical bills.

While your child is growing and thriving, you need to make sure that you are also taking care of yourself. In the next chapter, we will go through some self-care practices that you can put in place.

Chapter 9:

Self-Care for New Mothers

You are worth the quiet moment. You are worth the deeper breaths and you are worth the time it takes to slow down, be still, and rest. —Morgan Harper Nichols

When you have your first child, it is so easy to get caught up in looking after them, that you can completely forget to look after yourself as well. It may seem that it is not important, or that you are not a priority. But, did you know that your whole family will not be able to function if you are down and out? You may be able to get away with neglecting yourself for a short time, but eventually, it will catch up to you and the consequences can be relentless.

Many mothers even struggle to find the time just to take a shower! This is a basic need that needs to be done regularly, if not daily. Soon, moms will begin to feel insecure and uncared for. That is why I will be sharing some tips and advice on how to take care of yourself as a new mother.

Physical Self-Care Practices

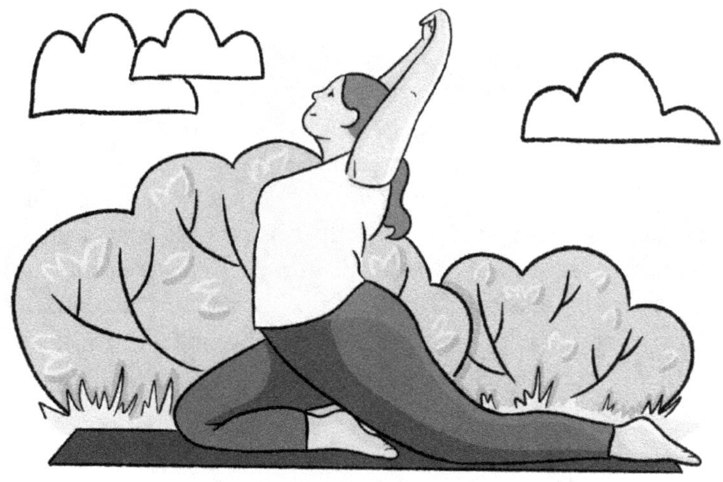

One of the most common areas where mothers fail to take care of themselves in the early stages of motherhood is through nutrition. This is usually followed closely by rest, exercise, and "me-time."

Your baby will not be eating solids yet, so you might struggle to find the time or motivation to make proper, nutritious meals. But remember that taking care of a baby is hard work and will take its toll on your body. Because of this, you need all the fuel and nutrition that you can get. If you are a breastfeeding mom, you will need to factor in the amount of calories and nutrients your body is burning through and these would need to be accounted for and replaced in order for your body to also get what it needs. Breastfeeding moms should drink plenty of water and try to eat protein at every meal. You can also continue to take your pregnancy vitamins throughout your breastfeeding journey to ensure that you are getting all the support that your body needs.

Catching up on rest is also a key part of practicing self-care. Now, I know all too well that this is easier said than done. But, you have to put time aside to sleep when your baby sleeps and to rest as much as possible.

This is especially true in the early days when your body has just gone through a lot during the birthing process, and your baby isn't sleeping through the night. You cannot possibly function on minimal sleep for months on end so put aside the chores and grab a blanket and pillow! If your baby is very demanding, or if you cannot bring yourself to sleep if you know there are things to be done, then don't be scared to call on a family member or close friend to help you out while you rest. Even a 20-minute nap can do wonders.

Start your day as if you were going to the office, or out with friends. What this means is that it can help your mindset immensely if you have a morning routine and get ready for the day as if it were an important day out. During the 2020 pandemic, multiple discussions showed that those who stayed in pajamas all day and didn't put in the effort were more likely to feel symptoms of depression than those who dressed up and had a routine in the morning. The first two weeks can be an exception to this rule as you will most likely be recovering from the birthing process.

Emotional Well-Being and Mental Health

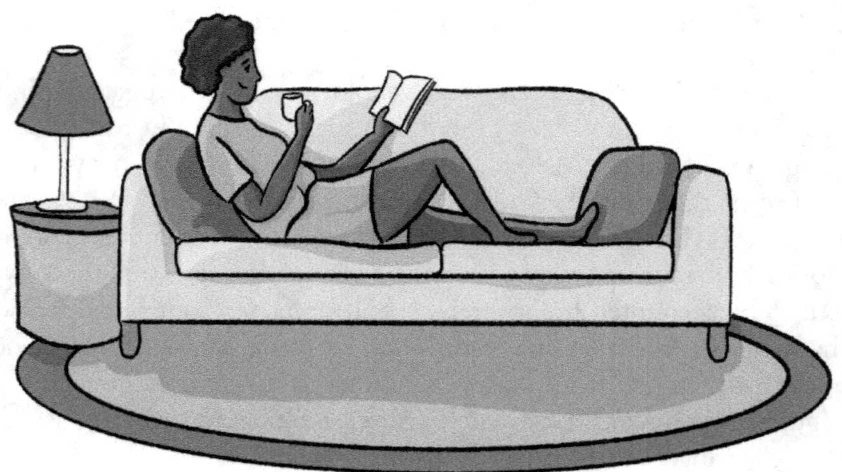

While mood swings during pregnancy can be totally normal and no cause for concern, these should not carry over into the post-partum period. It is normal to experience a few "off" days here and there, but if you feel down every single day for an extended period of time, then this could mean that there is something more serious going on and that you are experiencing symptoms of postpartum depression or even anxiety.

All moms will experience a dip in their mood a couple of days following the birth as their hormone levels will be changing again and their bodies will readjust to the new situation. This is usually what is referred to as the "baby blues." However, postpartum depression goes much deeper than this.

Research shows that one in five moms suffer from postpartum depression (Osbourne & Standeven, 2019). This is quite an alarming number of moms! Some of the most common signs include irritability, extreme fatigue, insomnia, intrusive or harmful thoughts, and deep levels of anxiety and sadness. If you experience these symptoms for more than two weeks, you should go see your healthcare provider as soon as possible. If left untreated for too long, postpartum depression can linger and will even stick around for a couple of years. It is best to get it seen as soon as possible so that you can enjoy your motherhood journey to the fullest.

In Summary

Being a new mother can be one of the hardest journeys that you will ever have to embark on. It's vital that you give yourself lots of grace and compassion. In all likelihood, you will be your own worst critic and you will make yourself feel guilty about all the things that you are doing wrong. I've found that moms experience this the most in the first month or two before babies can show signs of positive emotions, such as smiling or laughing. It is difficult for moms to know if they are doing a good enough job if the baby just cries and sleeps all the time. As adults, this pattern would indicate to us that something is wrong. But hang in there, that is all that your baby knows how to do at this stage and it does not at all reflect their happiness levels. Soon your baby will start smiling, babbling, and giggling, and you will be able to see their little personality developing right before your eyes. Remember that you are the best parent for them. You are their parent and no one else will do a better job at it than you can.

Your baby will grow so quickly and within the blink of an eye, they will be a couple of years old. Tracking their achievements and documenting their memories will be covered in the next chapter.

Chapter 10:

Celebrating Milestones and Cherishing Memories

The first steps that baby takes are into your heart. —Unknown

Looking back on your journey, you will realize that a lot has happened and many memories were made. In the moment, this might have felt like the longest few months of your life; but looking back, you will notice how quickly this went and you might even feel regretful that you didn't take enough time to celebrate each milestone or memory. This is not only about celebrating your child, but it is also about celebrating and appreciating you as a parent and all of the sacrifices that you have made to get the child to where they are today.

Documenting and Capturing Memories

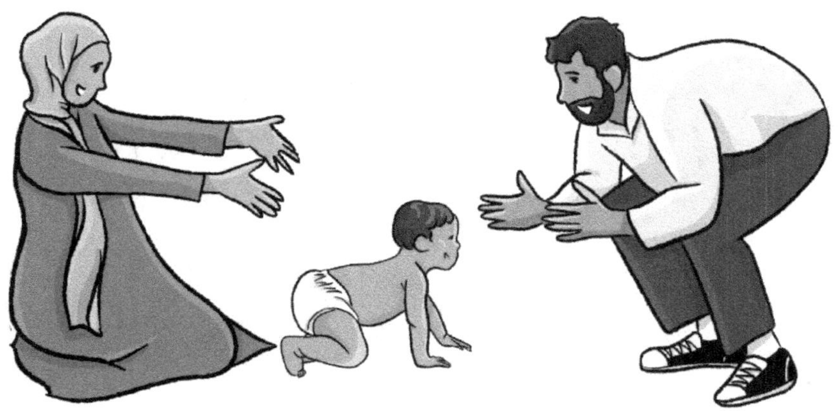

Baby journals and record books are the best way of capturing your baby's first year of life and tracking down the little memories that will easily slip our minds, such as the first food that your baby tasted, or the weight that they gained.

You can either buy an existing record book that you can fill out and glue photographs in, or you can make one from scratch. These also come in digital or print-out forms.

Try to fill in the book as you go along as you will forget or miss out on details the further away from the event you go. It is best to keep the book in an easily accessible place so that you can quickly note down the memory. You can also go through your photographs and select the ones that are dear to you and that you want to keep alive in memory. Think of any souvenirs or keepsakes that you think your child (or you) might be happy to see again twenty years down the line. Your creativity and sentimentality are key when it comes to tracking your baby's life.

A Walk Down Milestone Lane

Your baby's first year of life will be filled with precious memories and groundbreaking developments. These are the types of milestones that you would want to remember:

- first smile

- giggles

- first time sleeping through the night

- crawling

- waving

- clapping

- eating solids

- standing

- first steps

- first words

- any character traits that are unique to your baby

These are all moments that you will remember and cherish for years to come. Take a moment to reflect on each of these. If you are reading this before your baby is born, then reflect on what you want to feel in those moments and what you would like to do to be able to document these and remember them. If you have already gone through these milestones with your baby, then take a moment to reflect on each memory that you have of these incredible firsts.

First Birthday

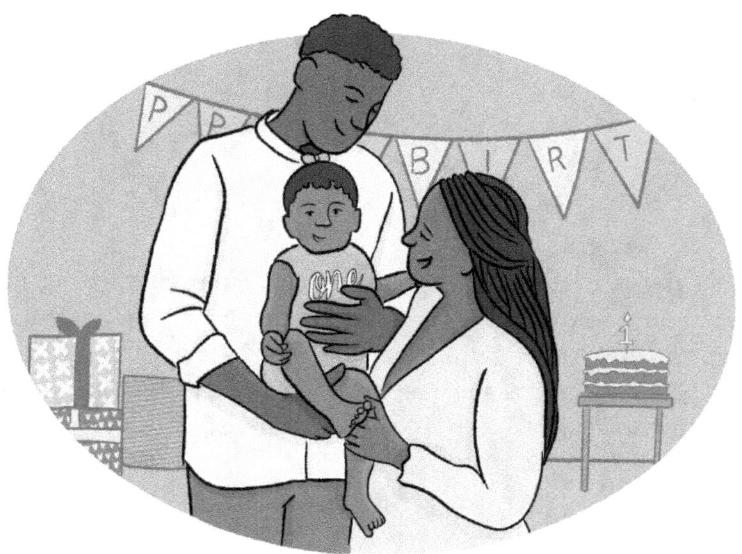

Congratulations! You have made it to your child's first birthday! There will be much to celebrate including the fact that you made it through the first year of your child's life! In essence, you made it through your first year as a parent. This is definitely a cause worthy of celebrating.

Take this opportunity to decide how you want to spend the day and how you want to make it unique and special for your child and yourself.

Some parents start a photo collage to be mounted on the wall of their child on their first birthday and every year to follow. Others may plant a shrub and watch it grow alongside their child. The possibilities are endless. What matters is that you do something special to commemorate all of your achievements and the time to come in further bonding, molding, and growing with your child.

Conclusion

Having a baby is a life-changing experience. Unless you have heaps of resources and help, you (along with your partner) will be dedicating your time to raising and looking after your little one. This can feel like a huge mountain of a task and a big responsibility. After all, you are raising a little human who will play a part in the future of your country, or even the world.

This book will help to guide and prepare you for what is to come in an otherwise overwhelming and unsure period in your life. By being prepared, you will be able to spend more time cherishing the moments that matter and loving the journey with your baby. It cannot be emphasized often enough that time will go by very quickly! Within a blink of an eye, your child will be starting school. That is why I want to set you up to enjoy every moment so that you can look back on the first few months, or even years, of your child's life and have no regrets about having missed out or been too stressed to fully enjoy them.

Parenting is not about being the perfect parent or raising a perfect child, this would set unrealistic expectations. But, it is about embracing the flaws and imperfections, learning from them, and working on them as a family. Every family is unique and comparison can be a killer. Instead of focusing on what others are doing, focus on nurturing your child and unlocking the potential that is unique to them.

I hope that this book will serve you throughout your parenting journey. I hope that you will find laughter in the good times, support in the bad times, and advice in the trying times. If you have found that this book has been of use to you, then why not pay it forward by gifting it to a friend or loved one who is about to embark on the parenthood journey? Leaving a review is also a great way to let others know what has helped you.

Above all, enjoy these next few months with your little one, and remember that you are doing a great job!

Keeping the Parenting Game Alive

As a parent, you have all the necessary tools to give your child the best. Now, it's time to help other young mothers find the same invaluable guidance you have.

You can share your honest opinion of this book on Amazon. This way, you'll show other parents where they can find the information they need and inspire them to pursue their passion for parenting newborns.

Your contribution is invaluable and plays a crucial role in the journey of newborn parenting. Let's share our knowledge and help each other.

Use the QR code below to leave your review on Amazon.

Appendix

√	**Furniture for Your New Baby**
	Crib
	Crib mattress
	Bassinet (optional)
	Rocking chair or glider
	Changing table with pad
	Chest of drawers of other clothes storage option
	Hanging or wall shelves
√	**Soft Items for Your New Baby**
	Waterproof crib mattress pad (1–3)
	Fitted crib sheets (2–4)
	Waterproof pad for bassinet (1–3, optional)
	Fitted bassinet sheets (2–4, optional)
	Changing table pad covers (2–4)

Swaddle blankets (2–4)

Receiving blankets (2–4)

Nursing pillow

Burp cloths (10–12)

Bibs (4–8)

Hooded bath towels (4–8)

Wash cloths (8–12)

Blackout curtains (optional)

√ **Clothing for Your New Baby**

Onesies (4–8)

Pajamas, sleepers, or sleeping sacks (4–8)

One-piece outfits (4–8)

Shirts that secure at the bottom (4–8)

Leggings or stretchy pants (4–8)

Dresses (4–8, optional)

Sweater or jacket

Socks or booties (4–8 pairs)

Hat with brim

√	
	Knit hat or cap
	Bunting bag or snowsuit
	Mittens
	Special outfit
√	**Feeding, Diapering, and Bathing Your New Baby**
	Bottles (8–10 each of 4 oz. and 6 oz.)
	Bottle nipples (8–10 each of 4 oz. and 6 oz.)
	Breast pump
	Milk storage bags or containers
	Bottle warmer
	Formula
	Bottle brush
	Bottle sterilizer
	Bottle drying rack
	Diaper bag
	Diapers (2–3 large boxes newborn size; 6–10 dozen cloth diapers; 6–8 diaper covers)
	Wipes (2–3 large boxes)

	Rash cream
	Diaper pail and liners
	Infant bathtub
	Bath caddy for toys and supplies
	Baby bath wash and shampoo
	Bath visor (optional)
	Baby lotion (optional)
	Soft-bristle hairbrush
	Infant nail clippers
	Pacifiers (4–6, optional)
√	**Miscellaneous Items for Your New Baby**
	Rear-facing infant car seat
	Stroller
	Infant swing (optional)
	Infant bouncer or stationary seat (optional)
	Portable crib (optional)
	Baby monitor
	Play mat for tummy time

	Age-appropriate toys
√	Outlet covers and other baby proofing items
	Toy bin
	Night light
	Mobile (optional)
	Music player (optional)
	Storage bins
	Closet organizer
	Drawer organizers
	Bathtub organizer or corner shelf
	Bottle organizer for kitchen storage
	Wearable baby carrier (optional)
	Sunscreen
	Gentle laundry detergent
	Bulb syringe
	Baby thermometer
	Teethers
√	**Just for You**

	Nipple cream
	Nursing bra
	Nursing pads
	Comfortable, loose-fitting clothing
	Nursing blankets or coverups
	Journal

About the Author

Nicole Stanton is a passionate author and dedicated mother with a wealth of personal experience in caring for newborns. Born and raised in the picturesque city of Colchester, Vermont, Nicole has always had a deep connection to her community and a strong desire to support and guide fellow parents on their journey. With four beautiful children—three boys and a girl—Nicole understands firsthand the joys, challenges, and rewards of raising a family. Her personal experiences have shaped her perspective and fueled her determination to provide valuable resources to new parents.

Nicole's journey as a mother has been marked by resilience and strength. She has faced and overcome numerous obstacles, including postpartum depression and breast cancer. These experiences have not only deepened her empathy and compassion for others but have also inspired her to share her knowledge and insights to help other parents navigate similar challenges.

The greatest triumph in Nicole's life came with the birth of her youngest child. Born with leukemia, the tiny fighter faced immense hurdles from the start. Nicole's unwavering love and determination, coupled with the support of her family and medical professionals, guided her child through a courageous battle against the disease. Witnessing her child's resilience and ultimate victory has fueled Nicole's passion for advocating for the health and well-being of newborns.

In her book, *The Newborn Parenting Guide (Made Easy): The Comprehensive Newborn Parenting Resource*, Nicole draws upon her personal experiences as a mother, her journey as an overcomer, and her unwavering commitment to her children's welfare. With proven methods, practical advice, and a clear-cut path toward mastering parenthood, Nicole empowers new parents to achieve better sleep, promote the health and wellness of their newborns, and navigate the challenges of early parenthood with confidence. Nicole's book serves as a beacon of hope and a comprehensive resource for parents seeking guidance and support in caring for their newborns. Through her writing, she aims to provide practical solutions, share her personal triumphs and challenges, and inspire parents to embrace the joys and responsibilities of parenthood.

Nicole resides in Scottsdale, Arizona, with her loving husband, John, to whom she has been happily married since 2014. Together, they continue to cherish their children and embody the spirit of resilience and unwavering love. Nicole Stanton's personal journey, filled with both triumphs and trials, has shaped her into an empathetic and knowledgeable resource for parents. Through her book and her own life experiences, she offers guidance, inspiration, and a message of hope to all those embarking on the incredible adventure of caring for newborns.

References

AAD. (n.d.). *How to treat diaper rash*. American Academy of Dermatology Association. https://www.aad.org/public/everyday-care/itchy-skin/rash/treat-diaper-rash

All4kids. (2021, August 14). *Bonding activities for parent and child*. Children's Bureau. https://www.all4kids.org/news/blog/bonding-activities-for-parent-and-child/

Amount and schedule of formula feedings. (2022, May 16). Healthy Children. https://www.healthychildren.org/English/ages-stages/baby/formula-feeding/Pages/Amount-and-Schedule-of-Formula-Feedings.aspx

Arnon, I. (2023). Starting big: Why is learning a language harder for adults than for children? *Frontiers for Young Minds, 11*. https://doi.org/10.3389/frym.2023.1011546

Babies' warning signs. (n.d.). Nationwide Children's Health. https://www.nationwidechildrens.org/family-resources-education/family-resources-library/babies-warning-signs

Baby first-aid kit guide. (n.d.). Children's Colorado. https://www.childrenscolorado.org/conditions-and-advice/parenting/parenting-articles/baby-first-aid-kit/

Baby Gooroo. (2019, March 2). *10 benefits of skin-to-skin contact*. Baby Gooroo. https://babygooroo.com/articles/10-benefits-of-skin-to-skin-contact

Barth, L. (2020, September 29). *How to bottle-feed a baby*. Healthline. https://www.healthline.com/health/baby/how-to-bottle-feed-a-baby#positions

BetterHealth (2019, September 30). *Child development (1)- Newborn to three months.* Better Health. https://www.betterhealth.vic.gov.au/health/HealthyLiving/child -development-1-newborn-to-three-months

Bilich, K. (2005, October 3). *Your step-by-step guide to bottle-feeding.* Parents. https://www.parents.com/baby/feeding/bottlefeeding/your- step-by-step-guide-to-bottlefeeding/

Blackman, K. (2020, May 29). *The complete nursery essentials checklist for new parents.* Newton Baby. https://www.newtonbaby.com/blogs/nursery/nursery-essentials

Blackman, K. (2023, January 21). *Bassinet vs. crib: What's the difference and which one is best for you.* Newton Baby. https://www.newtonbaby.com/blogs/nursery/bassinet-vs-crib

Blaker, K. (2022, February 12). *Child equipment safety for your baby, toddler, & preschooler.* Today's Family Magazine. https://www.todaysfamilymagazine.com/2022/02/12/294982/c hild-equipment-safety-for-your-baby-toddler-preschooler

Blankenship, J. (2022, April 15). *Ready to stop co-sleeping?* Baby Sleep Made Simple. https://www.babysleepmadesimple.com/how-to-stop- co-sleeping/

Bosshardt, G. (2023, October 23). *When can I sleep train my baby?* Intermountain Health. https://intermountainhealthcare.org/blogs/when-can-i-sleep- train-my-baby

Brandwein, S. (2020, September 29). *How to make a smooth transition from co- sleeping to crib.* Moshi. https://www.moshikids.com/articles/transition-from-co- sleeping-to-crib/

Bringing baby home: Tips for the transition. (n.d.). All About Women MD. https://www.allaboutwomenmd.com/knowledge- center/bringing-baby- home.html#:~:text=Getting%20Home&text=To%20increase%2 0your%20odds%20of

Bringing your baby home (for parents). (2022, June 8). Nemours Kids Health. https://kidshealth.org/en/parents/bringing-baby-home.html

Brown, T. (2022, March 9). *What to do when your baby has gas.* WebMD. https://www.webmd.com/parenting/baby/features/infant-gas

Buckley, A. (2020, July 12). *How to create a calm nursery for baby to sleep better.* Mama Mio. https://www.mamamio.com/blog/babies/how-to-create-calming-nursery/

Caring for Kids. (2021, August). *Your newborn: Bringing baby home.* Caring for Kids. https://caringforkids.cps.ca/handouts/pregnancy-and-babies/bringing_baby_home

Carter, M. (2023, August 11). *This is how often you should be bathing your newborn.* Parents. https://www.parents.com/baby/all-about-babies/heres-a-reason-to-skip-babys-bath-tonight/

Cassels, T. (2020, October 26). *The importance of partner support.* Evolutionary Parenting. https://evolutionaryparenting.com/importance-of-partner-support/

CDC. (2019, August 2). *Reasons to follow CDC's recommended immunization schedule.* Centers for Disease Control and Prevention. https://www.cdc.gov/vaccines/parents/schedules/reasons-follow-schedule.html

CDC. (2020a, March 31). *NIOSH training for nurses on shift work and long work hours.* Centers for Disease Control and Prevention. https://www.cdc.gov/niosh/work-hour-training-for-nurses/longhours/mod3/08.html

CDC. (2020b, February 24). *Feeding from a bottle.* Centers for Disease Control and Prevention. https://www.cdc.gov/nutrition/infantandtoddlernutrition/bottle-feeding/index.html

CDC. (2020c, February 24). *What to expect while breastfeeding.* Centers for Disease Control and Prevention. https://www.cdc.gov/nutrition/InfantandToddlerNutrition/breastfeeding/what-to-expect.html

CDC. (2020d, February 24). *When, what, and how to introduce solid foods.* Centers for Disease Control and Prevention. https://www.cdc.gov/nutrition/infantandtoddlernutrition/foods -and-drinks/when-to-introduce-solid- foods.html#:~:text=Your%20child%20can%20begin%20eating

CDC. (2023, March 21). *Newborn breastfeeding basics.* Centers for Disease Control and Prevention. https://www.cdc.gov/nutrition/infantandtoddlernutrition/breast feeding/newborn-breastfeeding-basics.html

Chatterjee, T. (2023, August 4). *Emergency care for 10 common injuries for children.* First Cry Parenting. https://parenting.firstcry.com/articles/first-aid-for-11-common- injuries-in-kids/

Chelsea. (2020, March 5). *Baby organization and nursery organization tips.* Two Twenty-One. https://www.twotwentyone.net/baby- organization/

Chen, J. (2021, March 19). *Nursery checklist: The essential items.* The Bump. https://www.thebump.com/a/creating-a-nursery

Child Mind Institute. (2023, February 23). *Complete guide to developmental milestones.* Child Mind Institute. https://childmind.org/guide/parents-guide-to-developmental- milestones/

Christiano, D. (2023, February 7). *Baby feeding schedule: A guide to the first year.* Healthline. https://www.healthline.com/health/parenting/baby-feeding- schedule#schedule-by-age

Cleveland Clinic. (2022a, July 13). *Infant sleep regression: What parents need to know.* Cleveland Clinic. https://health.clevelandclinic.org/the-4- month-sleep-regression-what-parents-need-to-know/

Cleveland Clinic. (2022b, March 4). *Why your baby needs tummy time.* Cleveland Clinic. https://health.clevelandclinic.org/3-benefits-of- tummy-time-for-newborns-how-to-do-it-safely

Cleveland Clinic. (n.d.). *Breastfeeding: How to start, benefits & common concerns.* Cleveland Clinic. https://my.clevelandclinic.org/health/articles/5182-breastfeeding

CMC Fresno. (2022, December 15). *When and how to sleep train your baby.* Children's Medical Centers of Fresno. https://cmcfresno.com/blog/when-and-how-to-sleep-train-your-baby/

Colic relief tips for parents. (2022, April 25). Healthy Children. https://www.healthychildren.org/English/ages-stages/baby/crying-colic/Pages/Colic.aspx

Colic relief tips for parents. (2022, April 25). Healthy Children. https://www.healthychildren.org/English/ages-stages/baby/crying-colic/Pages/Colic.aspx#:~:text=If%20you

Common worries and fears for parents. (2023, August 25). Pregnancy, Birth & Baby. https://www.pregnancybirthbaby.org.au/common-worries-and-fears-for-parents#:~:text=It%20is%20normal%20to%20feel

Consumer Guide. (2006, February 24). *Baby equipment safety tips.* How Stuff Works. https://lifestyle.howstuffworks.com/family/parenting/babies/how-to-buy-baby-equipment.htm

Coping with sleepless nights. (n.d.). Tommys. https://www.tommys.org/pregnancy-information/after-birth/coping-sleepless-nights

CPSC. (2016, January 8). *Safe sleep – Cribs and infant products.* Consumer Product Safety Commission. https://www.cpsc.gov/SafeSleep

Davies, I. (2021, October 29). *88 baby first steps quotes.* Find Your Mom Tribe. https://findyourmomtribe.com/baby-first-steps-quotes/

de Bellefonds, C. (2022, October 19). *Have a gassy baby? 13 ways to relieve infant gas.* What to Expect. https://www.whattoexpect.com/first-year/care/gassy-baby/#:~:text=Try%20the%20colic%20carry

Desitin. (n.d.). *How to prevent diaper rash in 3 easy steps.* Desitin. https://www.desitin.com/preventing-diaper-rash/how-to-prevent-diaper-rash

Developmental milestones: 0 to 6 months. (n.d.). Nationwide Children's Hospital. https://www.nationwidechildrens.org/family-resources-education/health-wellness-and-safety-resources/helping-hands/developmental-milestones-0-to-6-months

Different stages of breastmilk composition. (2019, January 1). NeoLacta Lifesciences. https://neolacta.com/blogs/different-stages-of-breastmilk-composition/

8 baby teething comfort tips every parent needs to know. (n.d.). Pediatric Dentistry of Burke Virginia. https://pediatricdentistryofburke.com/8-baby-teething-comfort-tips-every-parent-needs-to-know/

Elizabeth. (2023, September 15). *40 toddler & baby eating quotes you'll love.* Shoestring Baby. https://shoestringbaby.com/quotes-about-kids-eating-food/

Family Doctor. (2018, March 12). *Recognizing newborn illnesses.* Family Doctor. https://familydoctor.org/recognizing-newborn-illnesses/

FHS. (2018). *Parenting Series 2 - Responsive Care Bonding with Your Baby.* Family Health Service. https://www.fhs.gov.hk/english/health_info/child/13040.html

5 important baby exercises and 8 Important massages for your baby. (2021, February 23). Super Baby. https://www.superbabyonline.com/5-important-baby-exercises-8-important-massages-baby/

Garone, S. (2019, September 26). *Sleep consultants tell us how to survive the newborn days.* Healthline. https://www.healthline.com/health/sleep-consultants-share-tips-for-new-parents#The-Dos

Garoo, R. (2014, April 15). *6 essential tips on how to massage your baby.* Mom Junction. https://www.momjunction.com/articles/massage-baby_002856/

Gowmon, V. (n.d.). *Inspiring quotes on child learning and development.* Vince Gowmon. https://www.vincegowmon.com/inspiring-quotes-on-child-learning-and-development/

Gruber, B. (2020, January 7). *Newborn checklist: Everything you need before your baby arrives.* Today's Parent. https://www.todaysparent.com/checklists/newborn-checklist/

Gummer, A. (n.d.). *The role of play for newborn the child development: Playing at 0-6 months.* The Genius of Play. https://thegeniusofplay.org/genius/expert-advice/articles/the-role-of-play-for-newborn-child-development.aspx

Harper Nichols, M. (n.d.). *25 self-care quotes for moms and women.* But First, Joy. https://butfirstjoy.com/25-self-care-quotes-for-moms/

Harris, N. (2023, August 26). *A new parent's guide to estimating how many diapers you need and what they'll cost.* Parents. https://www.parents.com/parenting/money/saving/save-money-and-build-a-diaper-stockpile/

Harris, W. (2017, June 12). *5 design principles for a peaceful nursery.* Babyation. https://blog.babyation.com/5-design-principles-peaceful-nursery/

HealthPartners. (2020, July 20). *Why are vaccine schedules important for children?* Health Partners Blog. https://www.healthpartners.com/blog/importance-of-childhood-vaccine-schedules/

Higuero, V. (2020, June 18). *How to choose a pediatrician: 7 things to consider.* Healthline. https://www.healthline.com/health/childrens-health/how-to-choose-a-pediatrician#questions-to-ask

Holloway, C. (2022, July 13). *Infant sleep regression: What parents need to know.* Cleveland Clinic. https://health.clevelandclinic.org/the-4-month-sleep-regression-what-parents-need-to-know/

National Safety Council. (n.d.). *Home and community overview.* National Safety Council. https://injuryfacts.nsc.org/home-and-community/home-and-community-overview/introduction/

Hopper, A. (2023, July 31). *Find Your Mantra Momma: A New Mom's Guide to Conquering Postpartum, Anxiety, and all the Chaos That Comes From Childbirth*. Independently published.

How to choose the right doctor for your baby. (n.d.). Health Partners. https://www.healthpartners.com/care/everyday/kids-health/choosing-a-doctor-for-your-baby/

How to emotionally prepare for parenthood? (2021, April 26). Dadsnet. https://www.thedadsnet.com/how-to-emotionally-prepare-for-parenthood/

How to prepare your older children for a new baby. (2019, October 4). Healthy Children. https://www.healthychildren.org/English/ages-stages/prenatal/Pages/Preparing-Your-Family-for-a-New-Baby.aspx

Immunization schedule (for parents). (2018). Nemours Kids Health. https://kidshealth.org/en/parents/immunization-chart.html

Itzy Ritzy. (2020, October 1). *13 baby organization ideas & home storage tips*. Itzy Ritzy. https://www.itzyritzy.com/blogs/news/13-baby-organization-tips-to-help-simplify-life

Jain, S. (2023, August 6). *How often and how much should your baby eat?* American Academy of Pediatrics. https://www.healthychildren.org/English/ages-stages/baby/feeding-nutrition/Pages/How-Often-and-How-Much-Should-Your-Baby-Eat.aspx

Jemisin, N. K. (n.d.). *Top 25 protecting children quotes*. A-Z Quotes. https://www.azquotes.com/quotes/topics/protecting-children.html

Johns Hopkins Medicine. (n.d.-a). *Breast milk is best*. Johns Hopkins Medicine. https://www.hopkinsmedicine.org/health/conditions-and-diseases/breastfeeding-your-baby/breast-milk-is-the-best-milk

Johns Hopkins Medicine. (n.d.-b). *New parents: Tips for quality rest*. Johns Hopkins Medicine.

https://www.hopkinsmedicine.org/health/wellness-and-prevention/new-parents-tips-for-quality-rest

Judy, K. R. (2019). *Early developmental milestones*. Pathways. https://pathways.org/all-ages/milestones/

Karp, H. (n.d.). *The 5 s's for soothing babies*. Happiest Baby EU. https://happiestbaby.eu/blogs/baby/the-5-s-s-for-soothing-babies

Kashtan, P. (2023, May 30). *Baby checklist: 56 baby essentials*. The Bump. https://www.thebump.com/a/checklist-baby-essentials

Kids Health. (2018). *Immunization schedule (for parents)*. Kids Health. https://kidshealth.org/en/parents/immunization-chart.html

Kirova, K. (2017, March 19). *The importance of partner support for new mothers*. Krasi Kirova. https://kirovapsychology.com.au/2017/03/19/partners-are-the-one-person-that-new-mothers-need-the-most/

KK Women's and Children's Hospital. (n.d.). *Developmental exercises for your baby: Rolling, sitting, crawling*. Health Xchange. https://www.healthxchange.sg/children/baby-0-24-months/development-exercises-for-baby-rolling-sitting-crawling

Klein, E. (2023, May 22). *Can you sleep train a newborn? Expert advice and insights*. My Sleeping Baby. https://mysleepingbaby.com/sleep-train-newborns/

Kotlen, M. (2021, April 5). *Starting your breastfed baby on solid foods*. Verywell Family. https://www.verywellfamily.com/how-to-introduce-solid-foods-while-breastfeeding-431799

Krieger, L. (2022, April 9). *First week at home with your newborn baby*. Baby Center. https://www.babycenter.com/baby/newborn-baby/newborn-baby_10345806

Lewis, R. (2020, June 18). *Using the 5 S's to soothe your baby*. Healthline. https://www.healthline.com/health/baby/5-s-baby#swaddle

March of Dimes. (n.d.-a). *Baby blues after pregnancy*. March of Dimes. https://www.marchofdimes.org/find-support/topics/postpartum/baby-blues-after-pregnancy

March of Dimes. (n.d.-b). *Learning your baby's cues*. March of Dimes. https://www.marchofdimes.org/find-support/topics/neonatal-intensive-care-unit-nicu/learning-your-babys-cues#:~:text=Cues%20are%20signals%20from%20your

Marcin, A., & Dix, M. (2023, September 29). *7 of the best baby formulas*. Healthline. https://www.healthline.com/health/baby/best-baby-formula

Marcin, A. (2019, July 31). *Baby wearing: Benefits, safety tips, how-to, carrier types & more*. Healthline. https://www.healthline.com/health/parenting/baby-wearing#benefits

Martinelli, K. (2023, October 16). *Choosing a sleep training method that works for your family*. Child Mind Institute. https://childmind.org/article/choosing-a-sleep-training-method-that-works-for-your-family/

Masters, M. (2022, December 14). *How to cut your baby's nails*. What to Expect. https://www.whattoexpect.com/first-year/baby-care/baby-care-101/trim-nails.aspx

Mayo Clinic. (2017). *Solid foods: How to get your baby started*. Mayo Clinic. https://www.mayoclinic.org/healthy-lifestyle/infant-and-toddler-health/in-depth/healthy-baby/art-20046200

Mayo Clinic. (2022, July 1). *Diaper rash - Diagnosis and treatment*. Mayo Clinic. https://www.mayoclinic.org/diseases-conditions/diaper-rash/diagnosis-treatment/drc-20371641

Morgan, A. (2022, September 19). *How to practice self-care during pregnancy*. Munchkin. https://www.munchkin.com/blog/practicing-prenatal-care-for-you-and-baby/

Moyer, K. (2021, February 10). *Self-soothing baby: Benefits, behaviors, and techniques by age*. Medical News Today. https://www.medicalnewstoday.com/articles/self-soothing-baby

Muller, M. (2019, April 24). *10 things you didn't know about starting baby on solids*. The Bump. https://www.thebump.com/a/starting-solids-fun-facts

Mustela. (n.d.). *Baby hair care: The complete parent's guide*. Mustela USA. https://www.mustelausa.com/blogs/mustela-mag/baby-hair-care-the-complete-parent-s-guide

NAEYC. (2019). *Good toys for young children by age and stage*. National Association for the Education of Young Children. https://www.naeyc.org/resources/topics/play/toys

Nail care of newborn babies. (n.d.). India Parenting. https://www.indiaparenting.com/nail-care-of-newborn-babies.html

Nash, H. (2023, May 23). *Creating a safe & comfortable sleep environment for your newborn*. Tell Me Baby. https://tellmebaby.com.au/baby/creating-a-safe-comfortable-sleep-environment-for-your-newborn/

NCT. (2022, July 22). *Tips to help your baby to sleep*. National Childbirth Trust. https://www.nct.org.uk/baby-toddler/sleep/tips-help-your-baby-sleep

Newborn illness - how to recognize. (2019). Seattle Children's Hospital. https://www.seattlechildrens.org/conditions/a-z/newborn-illness-how-to-recognize/

Newton, A. (2020, June 5). *5 Reasons Why Your Newborn Isn't Sleeping at Night*. Healthline. https://www.healthline.com/health/parenting/newborn-not-sleeping

NHLBI. (2022, June 15). *How sleep affects your health*. National Heart, Lung, and Blood Institute. https://www.nhlbi.nih.gov/health/sleep-deprivation/health-effects

NHTSA. (n.d.). *Car seats and booster seats*. U.S. Department of Transportation National Highway Traffic Safety Administration. https://www.nhtsa.gov/equipment/car-seats-and-booster-seats#find-compare-seats

NMWIC. (n.d.). *Alternative feeding methods.* New Mexico Department of Health WIC Services. https://www.nmwic.org/breastfeeding-your-baby/nursing-a-b-cs/alternative-feeding-methods/

Nurturing healthy sleep habits in newborns. (2023, June 7). Nurtured Foundation. https://nurturedfoundation.com/healthy-sleep/

OASH. (2021, February 22). *Getting a good latch.* Office on Women's Health. https://www.womenshealth.gov/breastfeeding/learning-breastfeed/getting-good-latch#4

Osborne, L., & Standeven, L. (2019). *Postpartum mood disorders: What new moms need to know.* John Hopkins Medicine. https://www.hopkinsmedicine.org/health/wellness-and-prevention/postpartum-mood-disorders-what-new-moms-need-to-know

Pampers. (2022, October 25). *Newborn baby essentials: The ultimate baby checklist.* Pampers. https://www.pampers.com/en-us/pregnancy/preparing-for-your-new-baby/article/newborn-baby-checklist

Parents. (2015, July 14). *22 moms share the real joys of parenthood.* Parents. https://www.parents.com/parenting/better-parenting/the-real-joys-of-being-a-mom/

Pelly, J. (2019, November 18). *How often should you bathe your baby?* Healthline. https://www.healthline.com/health/baby/how-often-should-you-bathe-a-newborn#newborn

Perkins, E. (n.d.). *35+ new mom quotes and words of encouragement for mothers.* Shutterfly. https://www.shutterfly.com/ideas/new-mom-quotes/

Porretto, D. (2023, July 7). *Sleep deprivation after baby.* Parents. https://www.parents.com/baby/new-parent/sleep-deprivation/how-to-get-sleep/

Porter, R. (2018, August 28). *10 facts you didn't know about breastfeeding.* Western Missouri Medical Center. https://wmmc.com/ten-facts-about-breastfeeding

Rajneesh, B. S. (n.d.). *Rajneesh Quote*. A-Z Quotes. https://www.azquotes.com/quote/540762

Ratnam, G. (2023, June 14). *A quote by anonymous*. Firstcry Parenting. https://parenting.firstcry.com/articles/sleeping-baby-quotes-40-adorable-quotes-about-your-little-ones-snooze/

RCH. (2008). *Kids health info: Safety: Poisoning prevention*. Royal Children's Hospital. https://www.rch.org.au/kidsinfo/fact_sheets/Safety_Poisoning_prevention/

RCH. (n.d.). *Safety: Backyards and playgrounds*. Royal Children's Hospital. https://www.rch.org.au/kidsinfo/fact_sheets/Safety_Backyards_and_playgrounds/

Ronald, A. (2019, September 10). *How and when do babies develop social skills?* National Childbirth Trust. https://www.nct.org.uk/baby-toddler/emotional-and-social-development/how-and-when-do-babies-develop-social-skills

Shibu, A. (2022, October 26). *11 tips to cope with postpartum sleep deprivation*. Mini Klub Parenting. https://parenting.miniklub.in/tips-to-cope-with-postpartum-sleep-deprivation/

SickKids. (2009, October 18). *Nursery equipment safety for newborn babies*. About Kids Health. https://www.aboutkidshealth.ca/Article?contentid=437&language=English

SickKids. (2019, January 7). *Babies: How can you tell if your baby is ill?* About Kids Health. https://www.aboutkidshealth.ca/Article?contentid=710&language=English

Sleep guide - how to create the ideal sleep environment for babies and kids. (n.d.). Rockin' Blinks. https://rockinblinks.com/sleep-guides/sleep-environment

SMA. (n.d.). *Becoming a mum? Here's how you can emotionally prepare for parenthood*. SMA Nutrition.

https://www.smababy.co.uk/pregnancy/how-to-emotionally-prepare-for-parenthood

Smith-Garcia, D. (2021, January 28). *How to soothe a teething baby at night: 9 tips and tricks.* Healthline. https://www.healthline.com/health/baby/how-to-soothe-a-teething-baby-at-night#medicine

Srakocic, S. (2018, December 7). *Diaper rash treatment tips: Home remedies and more.* Healthline. https://www.healthline.com/health/home-remedies-diaper-rash#check-diaper-size

Stanley, C. (2020, June 8). *35+ new mom quotes and words of encouragement for mothers.* Shutterfly. https://www.shutterfly.com/ideas/new-mom-quotes/

Stavoe Harm, L. (n.d.). *Birth quotes.* Before and after the Birth. https://www.beforeandafterthebirth.org/birth-quotes

Stephens, C. (2020, December 8). *Self-soothing baby: Techniques for helping baby settle.* Healthline. https://www.healthline.com/health/baby/self-soothing-baby#leave-in-crib

Stern, D. (2021, May 4). *How to stock baby clothes for the first month: 10 steps.* Wikihow. https://www.wikihow.life/Stock-Baby-Clothes-for-the-First-Month

Sunshine, P. (n.d.). *Give 'em some skin.* Stanford Medicine Children's Health. https://www.stanfordchildrens.org/en/health-topics/magazine/give-em-some-skin

Takai. (n.d.). *Reading a baby's cues.* Takai. https://www.takai.nz/find-resources/articles/reading-a-babys-cues/

Taylor, G. (2022, December 11). *Is emotional readiness necessary for good parenting: 5 tips to unlock the power of emotional readiness! - heads up mom.* Heads up Mom. https://headsupmom.com/is-emotional-readiness-necessary-for-good-parenting/

Taylor, M. (2021, July 26). *When your newborn's hair will grow in — and why it's falling out.* What to Expect.

https://www.whattoexpect.com/first-year/ask-heidi/newborn-hair.aspx

10 incredible facts about your baby's brain. (2016, October 14). Tops Day Nurseries. https://www.topsdaynurseries.co.uk/10-incredible-facts-babys-brain/

Tips for getting enough sleep with a newborn. (2022, October 24). Baptist Health. https://www.baptisthealth.com/blog/mother-and-baby-care/tips-for-getting-enough-sleep-with-a-newborn

Tips to avoid diaper rash. (n.d.). Nationwide Children's Hospital. https://www.nationwidechildrens.org/family-resources-education/family-resources-library/tips-to-avoid-diaper-rash

Torrisi, J. (2021, July 6). *How to stop co-sleeping: A step by step guide.* Little Ones. https://www.littleones.co/blog/how-to-stop-co-sleeping-a-step-by-step-guide

Treeby, M. (2023, May 23). *Coping with sleep regression - Get through your baby's sleep regression.* Pampers. https://www.smartsleepcoach.com/blog/sleep-problems/how-to-cope-with-sleep-regressions

UNICEF. (n.d.). *Skin-to-skin contact.* UNICEF Baby Friendly Initiative. https://www.unicef.org.uk/babyfriendly/baby-friendly-resources/implementing-standards-resources/skin-to-skin-contact/#:~:text=There%20is%20a%20growing%20body

Vacco-Bolanos, J. (2023, May 13). *150 new mom quotes just in time for your first Mother's Day.* Parade. https://parade.com/1098145/jessicavacco/new-mom-quotes/

VetWest. (2022, July 27). *Children and pets.* VetWest Veterinary Clinics. https://www.vetwest.com.au/pet-library/children-and-pets-family-safety-bringing-home-a-baby/

Vieyra, D. (2023, January 6). *5 inspiring birth stories from real moms.* Peanut. https://www.peanut-app.io/blog/birth-stories

Villines, Z. (2021, February 10). *Self-soothing baby techniques and tips.* Medical News Today. https://www.medicalnewstoday.com/articles/self-soothing-baby#techniques

Watson, S. (2022, December 6). *Baby maintenance: Baths, nails, and hair.* WebMD. https://www.webmd.com/parenting/baby/baths-hair-and-nails

WebMD. (2019). *Baby milestones: Your child's first year of development.* WebMD. https://www.webmd.com/parenting/baby/ss/slideshow-baby-milestones-first-year

WebMD. (2022, August 29). *How much sleep do children need?* WebMD. https://www.webmd.com/parenting/guide/sleep-children

WIC. (2019). *Breastfeeding basics.* United States Department of Agriculture WIC Breastfeeding Support. https://wicbreastfeeding.fns.usda.gov/BREASTFEEDING-BASICS

Wisner, W. (2022, November 29). *All the essentials you need for a newborn baby.* Verywell Family. https://www.verywellfamily.com/bare-necessities-basic-baby-needs-293962

Wong, C. (2023, February 26). *Creating a peaceful sleep environment for your baby.* The Asian Parent. https://sg.theasianparent.com/ab00028-sleep-environment-for-baby

Young, B. (2022, August 15). *Choosing the right baby formula: A guide.* Healthline. https://www.healthline.com/health/parenting/baby-formula-guide-how-to-choose-the-right-kind-for-your-kid#fa-qs

Youngblood, T. (2023, April 20). *Helping sleep-deprived moms; How to get better sleep.* Sleepme. https://sleep.me/post/sleep-deprived-moms

Your baby's nap schedule: How to nail it! (n.d.). Nested Bean. https://www.nestedbean.com/pages/baby-nap-schedules

Zintl, A., & Curran, E. (2023, August 4). *How to massage a baby.* Parents. https://www.parents.com/baby/care/newborn/how-to-massage-baby/

www.ingramcontent.com/pod-product-compliance
Lightning Source LLC
Chambersburg PA
CBHW051615250726

48653CB00004BA/1515